Your *Clinics* subscription just got better!

You can now access the FULL TEXT of this publication online at no additional cost! Activate your online subscription today and receive...

- Full text of all issues from 2002 to the present
- Photographs, tables, illustrations, and references
- Comprehensive search capabilities
- Links to MEDLINE and Elsevier journals

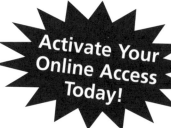

Plus, you can also sign up for E-alerts of upcoming issues or articles that interest you, and take advantage of exclusive access to bonus features!

To activate your individual online subscription:

1. Visit our website at **www.TheClinics.com**.

2. Click on "Register" at the top of the page, and follow the instructions.

3. To activate your account, you will need your subscriber account number, which you can find on your mailing label (note: the number of digits in your subscriber account number varies from six to ten digits). See the sample below where the subscriber account number has been circled.

This is your subscriber account number

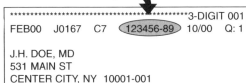

```
**************************************3-DIGIT 001
FEB00  J0167  C7  (123456-89)  10/00  Q: 1

J.H. DOE, MD
531 MAIN ST
CENTER CITY, NY  10001-001
```

4. That's it! Your online access to the most trusted source for clinical reviews is now available.

theclinics.com

ELSEVIER

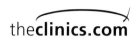

ORTHOPEDIC CLINICS

OF NORTH AMERICA

Revisiting Surface
Arthroplasty of the Hip

GUEST EDITORS
Paul E. Beaulé, MD, FRCSC
Michael Leunig, MD

April 2005 • Volume 36 • Number 2

SAUNDERS

An Imprint of Elsevier, Inc.
PHILADELPHIA   LONDON   TORONTO   MONTREAL   SYDNEY   TOKYO

W.B. SAUNDERS COMPANY
A Division of Elsevier Inc.

Elsevier Inc., 1600 John F. Kennedy Blvd., Suite 1800, Philadelphia, PA 19103-2899.

http://www.orthopedic.theclinics.com

ORTHOPEDIC CLINICS OF NORTH AMERICA   Volume 36, Number 2
April 2005   ISSN 0030-5898
Editor: Debora Dellapena   ISBN 1-4160-2745-9

The ideas and opinions expressed in *Orthopedic Clinics of North America* do not necessarily reflect those of the Publisher. The Publisher does not assume any responsibility for any injury and/or damage to persons or property arising out of or related to any use of the material contained in this periodical. The reader is advised to check the appropriate medical literature and the product information currently provided by the manufacturer of each drug to be administered to verify the dosage, the method and duration of administration, or contraindications. It is the responsibility of the treating physician or other health care professional, relying on independent experience and knowledge of the patient, to determine drug dosages and the best treatment for the patient. Mention of any product in this issue should not be construed as endorsement by the contributors, editors, or the Publisher of the product or manufacturers' claims.

Orthopedic Clinics of North America (ISSN 0030-5898) is published quarterly (For Post Office use only: Volume 36 issue 2 of 4) by Elsevier Inc. Corporate and editorial offices: Elsevier Inc., 1600 John F. Kennedy Blvd., Suite 1800, Philadelphia, PA 19103-2899. Accounting and circulation offices: 6277 Sea Harbor Drive, Orlando, FL 33887-4800. Periodicals postage paid at Orlando, FL 32862, and additional mailing offices. Subscription prices are $180.00 per year for (US individuals), $295.00 per year for (US institutions), $214.00 per year (Canadian individuals), $351.00 per year (Canadian institutions), $245.00 per year (international individuals), $351.00 per year (international institutions), $90.00 per year (US students), $123.00 per year (Canadian and international students). Foreign air speed delivery is included in all *Clinics* subscription prices. All prices are subject to change without notice. POSTMASTER: Send address changes to *Orthopedic Clinics of North America,* W.B. Saunders Company, Periodicals Fulfillment, Orlando, FL 32887-4800. **Customer Service: 1-800-654-2452 (US). From outside of the US, call 1-407-345-4000. E-mail: hhspcs@harcourt.com.**

Reprints. For copies of 100 or more, of articles in this publication, please contact the Commercial Reprints Department, Elsevier Inc., 360 Park Avenue South, New York, New York 10010-1710. Tel. (212) 633-3813 Fax: (212) 462-1935 e-mail: reprints@elsevier.com

Orthopedic Clinics of North America is covered in *Index Medicus, Cinahl, Excerpta Medica, and Cumulative Index to Nursing and Allied Health Literature.*

Printed in the United States of America.

GUEST EDITORS

PAUL E. BEAULÉ, MD, FRCSC, Assistant Clinical Professor, David Geffen School of Medicine at University of California Los Angeles; Joint Replacement Institute at Orthopaedic Hospital, Los Angeles, California

MICHAEL LEUNIG, MD, Associate Professor, Department of Orthopaedic Surgery, University of Berne, Inselspital, Berne, Switzerland

CONTRIBUTORS

HARLAN C. AMSTUTZ, MD, Director, Joint Replacement Institute at Orthopaedic Hospital, Los Angeles, California

JOHN ANTONIADES, MD, Joint Replacement Institute at Orthopaedic Hospital, Los Angeles, California

D.L. BACK, FRCS (Edin) (Orth), Research Fellow, The Melbourne Orthopaedic Group, Melbourne, Australia

J. BARE, MBBS, FRACS, FAOrthA, Consultant Orthopedic Surgeon, The Melbourne Orthopaedic Group, Melbourne, Australia

PAUL E. BEAULÉ, MD, FRCSC, Assistant Clinical Professor, David Geffen School of Medicine at University of California Los Angeles; Joint Replacement Institute at Orthopaedic Hospital, Los Angeles, California

MARTIN BECK, MD, Assistant Professor and Attending Orthopaedic Surgeon, Department of Orthopaedic Surgery, University of Berne, Inselspital, Berne, Switzerland

RUDI G. BITSCH, MD, Joint Replacement Institute at Orthopaedic Hospital, Los Angeles, California

HENDRIK BOSCH, FRCS, Visiting Fellow, Department of Orthopaedics and Trauma, Royal Gwent Hospital, Newport, Wales

JOHN G. BOWSHER, PhD, Orthopedic Research Center, Loma Linda University Medical Center, Loma Linda, California

IAN C. CLARKE, PhD, Professor of Orthopedic Research and Director, Orthopedic Research Center, Loma Linda University Medical Center, Loma Linda, California

KERRY COSTI, BA, Research Officer, Department of Orthopaedics and Trauma, Royal Adelaide Hospital, Adelaide, South Australia

KOEN A. DE SMET, MD, Hip Surgeon, Hipcentre, Jan Palfijn Hospital, Ghent; Director, Anca Clinic, Heusden, Belgium

VALENTIN DJONOV, MD, Associate Professor, Department of Anatomy, University of Berne, Inselspital, Berne, Switzerland

THOMAS DONALDSON, MD, Adjunct Professor of Orthopedics and Director, Joint Replacement Center, Loma Linda University Medical Center, Loma Linda, California

VINCENT A. FOWBLE, MD, Joint Replacement Institute at Orthopaedic Hospital, Los Angeles, California

REINHOLD GANZ, MD, Professor, Department of Orthopaedic Surgery, University of Berne, Inselspital, Berne, Switzerland

PATRIC GNEPF, Zimmer GmbH, Winterthur, Switzerland

STEPHEN E. GRAVES, PhD, FRACS, MBBS, Professor, Department of Medicine, University of Melbourne, Melbourne; Director, Department of Orthopaedics, Royal Melbourne Hospital, Parkville, Victoria, Australia

MICHAEL J. GRECULA, MD, Associate Professor, Department of Orthopaedics and Rehabilitation, University of Texas Medical Branch, Galveston, Texas

PETER GRIGORIS, FRCS, FACS, Honorary Professor, Department of Medical Engineering, School of Engineering, Design, and Technology, University of Bradford, Bradford, West Yorkshire, United Kingdom; Visiting Professor, 2nd Orthopaedic Department, University of Athens, Ag. Olga Hospital, Athens, Greece

RYAN HOKE, BS, Joint Replacement Institute at Orthopaedic Hospital, Los Angeles, California

DONALD W. HOWIE, PhD, FRACS, MBBS, Professor and Head, Department of Orthopaedics and Trauma, University of Adelaide and Royal Adelaide Hospital; Clinical Director, Orthopaedic and Trauma Service, Royal Adelaide Hospital, Adelaide, South Australia

MORTEZA KALHOR, MD, Attending Orthopaedic Surgeon, Iran University of Medical Sciences, Firouzgar Medical Center, Tehran, Iran

RETO KONRAD, Zimmer GmbH, Winterthur, Switzerland

MARTIN LAVIGNE, MD, FRCSC, Attending Orthopaedic Surgeon, Department of Orthopaedic Surgery, Hôpital Maisonneuve-Rosemont; Assistant Clinical Professor, Department of Surgery, University of Montreal, Montreal, Canada

MICHEL J. LE DUFF, MA, Clinical Research Coordinator, Joint Replacement Institute, Orthopaedic Hospital, Los Angeles, California

MICHAEL LEUNIG, MD, Associate Professor, Department of Orthopaedic Surgery, University of Berne, Inselspital, Berne, Switzerland

GERNOT LIEBENTRITT, Zimmer GmbH, Winterthur, Switzerland

ANASTASIOS K. LILIKAKIS, MD, Orthopaedic Surgeon, Athens, Greece

MARGARET A. McGEE, MPH, Senior Medical Scientist, Department of Orthopaedics and Trauma, University of Adelaide and Royal Adelaide Hospital, Adelaide, South Australia

SAM NASSER, MD, PhD, Associated Professor, Department of Orthopedics, Wayne State University School of Medicine and Department of Biomedical Engineering, Wayne State University College of Engineering, Detroit, Michigan

SEAN E. NORK, MD, Allgöwer Fellow, Arbeitsgemeinschaft fur Osteosynthesefragen North America; Associate Professor, Harborview Medical Center, Department of Orthopaedic Surgery, Seattle, Washington

KOSTANTINOS PANOUSIS, MD, Orthopaedic Surgeon, Athens Medical, Athens, Greece

GILLES PFANDER, Medical Student, Department of Orthopaedic Surgery, University of Berne, Inselspital, Berne, Switzerland

CLAUDE B. RIEKER, PhD, Tribology Director, Zimmer GmbH, Winterthur, Switzerland

PAUL ROBERTS, MA(Oxon), MB, FRCS, Consultant Orthopaedic Surgeon, Royal Gwent Hospital, Newport, Wales

MICHAEL SCHÄR, Medical Student, Department of Orthopaedic Surgery, University of Berne, Inselspital, Berne, Switzerland

ROLF SCHÖN, Zimmer GmbH, Winterthur, Switzerland

ALEXANDER SCHUH, MD, Orthopedic Clinic Wichernhaus, Schwarzenbruck, Germany

MING SHEN, Zimmer GmbH, Winterthur, Switzerland

A. J. SHIMMIN, MBBS, FRACS, FAOrthA, DipAnat, Consultant Orthopedic Surgeon, The Melbourne Orthopaedic Group, Melbourne, Australia

EDWIN P. SU, MD, Assistant Attending Orthopaedic Surgeon, Hospital for Special Surgery, New York, New York

TOMOKI TAKAHASHI, MD, Department of Orthopaedic Surgery, Kumamoto University of Medicine, Kumamoto City, Kumamoto Prefecture, Japan

RICHARD N. VILLAR, MS, FRCS, Consultant Orthopaedic Surgeon, Cambridge Hip and Knee Unit, BUPA Cambridge Lea Hospital, Cambridge, United Kingdom

SARAH L. VOWLER, MSc, Medical Statistician, Centre for Applied Medical Statistics, Department of Public Health and Primary Care, University of Cambridge, Cambridge, United Kingdom

CONTENTS

Metal-on-metal hip resurfacing, a significant recent development in hip arthroplasty, preserves proximal femoral bone stock, optimizes stress transfer to the proximal femur, and offers inherent stability and optimal range of movement. The results of hip resurfacing in the 1970s and 1980s were disappointing, and the procedure was largely abandoned by the mid-1980s. The renaissance of metal-on-metal articulations for total hip arthroplasty has enabled the introduction of new hip resurfacings, and many implant manufacturers have introduced such systems. Early results are encouraging, and complications commonly seen in the 1970s and 1980s, such as early implant loosening and femoral neck fracture, are rare. Background research and better understanding of implant failure suggest that current hip resurfacing technology has developed beyond that of an experimental procedure.

Large diameter metal-on-metal articulations may provide an opportunity for wear reduction in total hip implants because earlier studies have shown that the formation of a fluid film that completely separates the bearing surfaces is theoretically possible. In such a lubrication mode and under ideal conditions, there is theoretically no amount of wear. Studies have suggested that the two primary parameters controlling the lubrication mode are the diameter and the clearance of the articulation. The goal of the present study was to experimentally investigate the influence of these two parameters on the wear behavior of large diameter metal-on-metal articulations pertaining to resurfacing hip implants. The results of this in vitro investigation showed that longer running-in periods and higher amounts of running-in wear were associated with larger clearances.

to closely reproduce the normal anatomy of the proximal femur, surgeons performing this procedure need to take into consideration the underlying pathology that led to the degenerative changes. Consequently, choice of surgical approach and positioning of the implants may have a greater impact on implant survivorship and patient function than in standard hip replacement. This article presents case illustrations of different hip pathologies treated by surface arthroplasty of the hip.

Hip resurfacing arthroplasty is an old orthopedic concept that has undergone a resurgence of interest in the past decade. Because of the rapid increase in the number of procedures being performed, previously recognized complications have begun to recur. This article focuses on complications that are related to the hip resurfacing procedure such as femoral neck fractures, avascular necrosis, raised metal ion levels, and sound initial and durable long-term fixation of an all-metal monoblock cobalt/chrome acetabular component. Dislocation rates after resurfacing and other complications are briefly discussed.

This article describes a randomized clinical trial in young patients, comparing metal-on-metal cemented resurfacing hip replacement with cemented total hip replacement. The trial was stopped early, mainly because of a high incidence of failure of the cemented resurfacing acetabular component. The results reinforce the importance of clinical trials for evaluating the safety and efficacy of prosthesis designs before being used in a large cohort of patients. Although there may be advantages of resurfacing hip replacement, trials are also required to demonstrate it has a mid- to long-term success that reasonably approaches that of total hip replacement.

Hybrid metal-on-metal surface arthroplasty of the hip has recently been introduced, with a vast number of implants used in European countries including Belgium. This article presents results in 252 hips with a mean follow-up of 2.8 years. Using a tight press-fit with minimal cement mantle as the technique of femoral fixation, there have been only three failures. The main complications have been avascular necrosis of the femoral head and femoral neck fracture. In most cases, patients returned to a high functional level with no restrictions in their physical activity and were highly satisfied. Future refinements in surgical technique and instruments will make this procedure more accessible and reproducible for the surgeon.

The authors report preliminary results of an uncemented, hydroxyapatite-coated femoral implant for metal-on-metal hip resurfacing. The survival rate of 70 implants after at least 2 years follow-up was 98.6%, with an excellent clinical outcome. There have been no femoral fractures, aseptic loosening, or radiolucencies around the stem. Thinning of the femoral neck at the inferomedial cup-neck rim has been a frequent radiologic finding but with no clinical implication so far. Longer follow-up is needed to confirm the results.

FORTHCOMING ISSUES

RECENT ISSUES

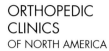

ORTHOPEDIC
CLINICS
OF NORTH AMERICA

ELSEVIER
SAUNDERS

Orthop Clin N Am 36 (2005) xiii – xiv

Preface

Revisiting Surface Arthroplasty of the Hip

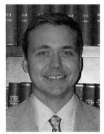
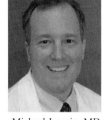

Paul E. Beaulé, MD, FRCSC   Michael Leunig, MD
Guest Editors

After the first "Symposium on Surface Arthro-plasty of the Hip," Marvin Steinberg [1], the *Ortho-pedic Clinics of North America* guest editor at the time, concluded "surface arthroplasty of the hip should be considered in the stage of evaluation and only performed by surgeons with considerable experience in hip reconstruction." In recent years, there has been a renaissance of surface arthroplasty of the hip with the re-introduction of metal-on-metal articulations in total hip arthroplasty. With the current success of modern total hip replacements, however, one might ask what the role of hip resurfacing for today's orthopedic surgeon should be. Will the intro-duction of metal-on-metal bearings significantly de-crease the failure rate previously experienced with the first generation of hip resurfacing? What factors will determine the successful outcome of this conservative prosthetic implant? These questions are what moti-vated us as guest editors to devote a second vol-ume on hip resurfacing entitled "Revisiting Surface Arthroplasty of the Hip."

The theoretic advantages of surface arthroplasty have not changed and include preservation of proximal femoral bone stock, optimization of stress transfer to the proximal femur, enhanced inherent stability, and optimal range of movement due to the large diameter of the articulation. As reviewed in this issue by Grigoris et al, failures that caused the

procedure to be largely abandoned by the mid-1980s were the consequences of inappropriate materials, poor implant design, inadequate instrumentation, and to some extent, an inherent problem with the procedure itself. Reiker et al, revealing a long expe-rience in metal-on-metal tribology, provides us with insight into the key factors determining the low wear rate of large-diameter metal-on-metal bearings. The article on design issues facing hip resurfacing implants by Clarke and associates is particularly interesting because the lead author was an engineer involved in the development of hip resurfacing in the late 1970s.

To date, the choice of surgical approach (posterior being most common) does not appear to have a significant impact on the clinical outcome; however, the impact of the posterior approach on the blood supply to the femoral head is relatively unknown and starting to be questioned. The articles by Nork et al and Lavigne et al bring to light important anatomic and biologic aspects of the proximal femur that have not been appreciated due to the predominance of stem-type designs in total hip replacements. The respect for the hip's soft tissue envelope, which is strived for by current hip arthroplasty surgeons, must also be integrated into hip resurfacing, which in turn will help minimize complications such as femoral neck fractures. Beaulé and Antoniades discuss some

0030-5898/05/$ – see front matter © 2005 Elsevier Inc. All rights reserved.
doi:10.1016/j.ocl.2005.02.003

orthopedic.theclinics.com

of these principles in addition to patient selection, which has served well other conservative procedures such as hip osteotomies. Shimmin and associates from Australia (another country where hip resurfacing has been embraced) provide us with a detailed review of potential complications specific to hip resurfacing. The article by Howie and associates, also from Australia, recognizes the value of randomized clinical trials in the evaluation of new technology.

The next four articles provide the reader with an overview of the clinical results of hip resurfacing. De Smet gives insight into patient function and clinical outcome based on large clinical series of more than 1000 cases. Lilikakis and associates discuss the early clinical results of cementless fixation on the femoral side. The last two clinical articles bring insight into challenging cases: Amstutz and associates discuss the arthritic hip secondary to childhood disorders and Grecula describes treating osteonecrosis of the hip. Finally, Fowble and associates continue to explore the applications of implant migration analysis in monitoring the long-term outcome of hip resurfacing.

To us, it is important to consider hip surface arthroplasty not as a substitute for total hip replacement, which works so well, but as an additional treatment option for the cohort of young and active patients in whom conventional replacement still provides mixed results. Combining surface arthroplasty in cases of early osteoarthritis caused by proximal femoral or acetabular abnormalities with surgical techniques to improve hip biomechanics appears to be a promising conservative treatment concept.

We enjoyed editing this issue and thank all of the authors for their time and effort. Moreover, we thank Debora Dellapena of the *Orthopedic Clinics of North America*, with whom it has been a pleasure to work.

Paul E. Beaulé, MD, FRCSC
Assistant Clinical Professor
David Geffen School of Medicine at
University of California Los Angeles
Los Angeles, CA, USA

Joint Replacement Institute at Orthopaedic Hospital
2400 S. Flower Street
Los Angeles, CA 90007, USA
E-mail address: pbeaule@laoh.ucla.edu

Michael Leunig, MD
Department of Orthopaedic Surgery
University of Berne, Inselspital
CH-3010 Berne, Switzerland
E-mail address: michael.leunig@balgrist.ch

Reference

[1] Steinberg ME. Summary and conclusions: symposium on surface replacement arthroplasty of the hip. Orthop Clin N Am 1982;13:895–902.

ORTHOPEDIC
CLINICS
OF NORTH AMERICA

Orthop Clin N Am 36 (2005) 125 – 134

The Evolution of Hip Resurfacing Arthroplasty

Peter Grigoris, FRCS[a,b,*], Paul Roberts, MA(Oxon), MB, FRCS[c],
Kostantinos Panousis, MD[d], Hendrik Bosch, FRCS[c]

[a]Department of Medical Engineering, School of Engineering, Design, and Technology, University of Bradford, Richmond Road,
Bradford, West Yorkshire BD7 1DP, UK
[b]2nd Orthopaedic Department, University of Athens, Ag. Olga Hospital, 142 33 N. Ionia, Athens, Greece
[c]Department of Orthopaedics and Trauma, Royal Gwent Hospital, Cardiff Road, Newport NP9 2UB, Wales
[d]Athens Medical, Distomou 5-7, 151 25 Marousi, Athens, Greece

Total hip replacement in its current format has proved very effective in late middle-aged and elderly patients, with survival rates in excess of 90% at 10 years [1]. When younger patients are reviewed, however, especially men younger than 55 years old, this survival figure drops to 80% at 10 years. This trend worsens by 16 years postoperatively, with reported survival figures as low as 33%. Hip resurfacing is being advocated as an alternative treatment for young and active patients with hip disease. Resurfacing is an attractive concept because it preserves proximal femoral bone stock, optimizes stress transfer to the proximal femur, and because of the large diameter of the articulation, offers inherent stability and optimal range of movement [2].

History

The concept of hip resurfacing is not new. Contemporary designs have evolved directly from the original mold arthroplasty introduced by Smith-Petersen in 1948 [3]. Despite being a hemiarthroplasty with no means of stable fixation to the femoral head, some survived for many years, although the outcomes were unpredictable. The first total resurfacing arthroplasty was developed by Charnley [4,5] in the early 1950s using a Teflon-on-Teflon bearing.

This implant was associated with high early failure that Charnley ascribed to avascular necrosis of the femoral head. Charnley subsequently recognized the poor wear characteristics of Teflon when he used it as the bearing of a total hip replacement.

In 1960, Townley [6] attempted hip resurfacing using a metal-on-polyurethane articulation that was also associated with catastrophic wear (Fig. 1). It was later replaced by a metal-on-polyethylene articulation.

In 1967, Muller [7,8] designed a metal-on-metal articulation. He implanted 18 surface replacements in young patients in addition to 35 stemmed prostheses (Fig. 2). Despite excellent early clinical results, Muller abandoned the use of the metal-on-metal articulation in favor of a metal-on-polyethylene articulation. Six of these all-metal articulations were revised after functioning for up to 25 years.

Gerard [9] introduced a bipolar metal-on-metal resurfacing in 1970. The system consisted of a Luck cup inserted into an Aufranc Vitallium cup (Howmedica Inc, Rutherford, NJ), with movement occurring between the prostheses and between the outer cup and the bony socket. In 1972, the Aufranc cup was substituted with a polyethylene cup in an attempt to decrease the friction between the two implants; however, the convex surface of the polyethylene component that articulated with the acetabulum wore rapidly and this combination was abandoned in 1975 in favor of a metal bipolar combination with a polyethylene inlay.

In Japan, Furuya [10] performed 13 hip resurfacings using a stainless steel acetabular component with a high density polyethylene (HDP) femoral compo-

* Corresponding author. Souidias 68, 115 21 Athens, Greece.
   E-mail address: p.grigoris@tellas.gr (P. Grigoris).

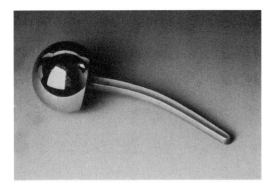

Fig. 1. The TARA femoral component originally designed as a femoral hemiresurfacing arthroplasty.

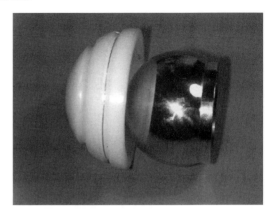

Fig. 3. Cemented hip resurfacing developed by Paltrinieri and Trentani in Italy. It had a thin-walled, all-polyethylene acetabular cup and a stainless steel femoral component with a 3-mm collar.

nent fixed with cement, then subsequently reversed the material combination, using a metal or ceramic femoral component. In 1972, Nishio [11] combined a Urist acetabular component with his own femoral component made from Vitallium; in 1975, they substituted the acetabular component with a polyethylene-lined cementless socket. Tanaka [12], in 1974, introduced a hybrid system with a cemented eccentric socket and a metal head.

Cemented hip resurfacings using polyethylene acetabular components and metal femoral components were implanted in 1971 by Paltrinieri and Trentani [13] in Italy (Fig. 3) and in 1974 by Freeman [14,15] in the United Kingdom. Freeman had earlier used a HDP femoral component and a metal acetabular component, but this was associated with rapid wear of the convex surface. In the same year in Germany, Wagner introduced a hip resurfacing (Fig. 4) that became widely used in Europe [16]. The acetabular components had a thickness of only 4 mm. Cobalt–chromium (Co-Cr) and ceramic femoral components were available, but head preparation was crude. Starting in 1976, a cementless alumina ceramic-on-ceramic resurfacing was used by Salzer [17] in Vienna but was soon abandoned because of high rates of early loosening.

In 1973 in the United States, Eicher and Capello [18] developed a cemented hip resurfacing using a metal femoral and a polyethylene acetabular component. The acetabular component was reinforced with a metal backing in 1982. In 1975, Amstutz [19,20] introduced the THARIES (total hip articular replacement using internal eccentric shells) at the University of California–Los Angeles. The prosthesis was cemented and consisted of a Co-Cr femoral component and an all-polyethylene acetabular component (Fig. 5). Both components were eccentric, with a maximum polyethylene thickness of 3.5 to

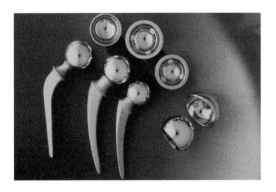

Fig. 2. Metal-on-metal hip prostheses introduced by Muller and Huggler in 1967. On the far right is a cementless hip resurfacing.

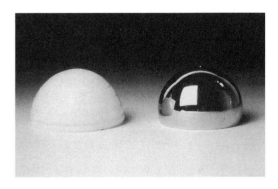

Fig. 4. Cemented metal-on-polyethylene resurfacing system introduced by Wagner in 1974.

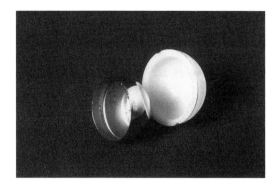

Fig. 5. The THARIES cemented resurfacing arthroplasty developed by Amstutz in 1975. It consisted of an eccentric Co-Cr femoral component articulating with an eccentric all-polyethylene acetabular cup. (*Courtesy of* H.C. Amstutz and P.E. Beaulé.)

5.5 mm. A plasma-sprayed metal-backed polyethylene acetabular component for use with cement was introduced in 1982 [21]. In 1983, Amstutz [21,22] implanted the first cementless resurfacing arthroplasty with a Ti-6Al-4V femoral component, modular ultra high molecular weight polyethylene acetabular liners, and pure titanium mesh porous backing. Initially, the sockets were hemispherical with screws, and later, the first chamfered cylinder socket with an interference fit was developed (Fig. 6). In 1988, Amstutz developed another porous-coated cementless system with a Co-Cr femoral component, a modular liner, and a Ti-6Al-4V hemispherical acetabular component. In 1989, Buechel and Pappas [23] introduced a cementless resurfacing system with a modular acetabular component and a titanium nitride ceramic-coated titanium alloy femoral component.

Modes of failure of first-generation resurfacings

The results of hip resurfacing in the 1970s and 1980s were disappointing, and the procedure was largely abandoned by the mid-1980s, with the exception of a small number of centers. The expectation that these prostheses would be easy to revise was not often fulfilled. Although proximal femoral bone stock was well maintained, there was often extensive destruction of the acetabulum. This destruction, partly a consequence of the excessive removal of bone required to accommodate the acetabular component and the cement mantle, was mainly due to periprosthetic osteolysis.

With our present knowledge, the first generation of metal-on-polyethylene resurfacings represents an excellent model of a high-wear–producing bearing. The large diameter of the articulation combined with thin polyethylene cups or liners led to accelerated wear and the production of large volumes of biologically active particulate debris, leading to bone loss and implant loosening. Because the implications of wear debris–induced osteolysis were not fully appreciated at the time, failure was attributed to other factors including avascular necrosis of the femoral head and acetabular component loosening due to high frictional torque. The high incidence of femoral neck fracture was also an issue.

Retrieval studies have not confirmed whether resurfacing of the femoral head leads to avascular necrosis. Howie et al [24] examined 72 failed Wagner resurfacings and concluded that there was viable bone in the femoral head and neck in most cases. The bone destruction was consistent with wear particle–induced osteolysis, not avascular necrosis. Similar findings have been reported by other investigators [18,25]. Freeman [26] argued that the major blood supply to the arthritic femoral head is through intraosseous vessels, not through the subsynovial anastomoses. Such intraosseous vessels would not be disrupted during the exposure and preparation of the femoral head. This may explain why avascular necrosis has not been proved to be a significant complication following hip resurfacing; however, the debate concerning the effect that resurfacing has on the blood supply of the femoral head continues.

The influence of the increased frictional torque, which is a consequence of the large diameter of the articulation, was addressed by Mai et al [27]. A relatively homogeneous group of 170 osteoarthritic

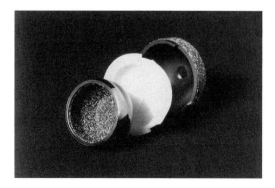

Fig. 6. The Porous Surface Replacement system introduced by Amstutz in 1983. The femoral head was a titanium alloy with sintered titanium fiber mesh. The modular acetabular cup consisted of a chamfered titanium alloy shell and a polyethylene liner. (*Courtesy of* H.C. Amstutz and P.E. Beaulé.)

patients who underwent a cemented THARIES resurfacing arthroplasty was studied. Hips were divided into three groups according to the diameter of the articulation. Using survivorship analysis, the investigators showed that despite higher frictional torque due to the increased diameter of the bearing surface and the increased average load, the larger prostheses survived significantly longer than the smaller ones. Stepwise covariate discriminant analysis indicated that the size of the bearing surface was the only factor that significantly affected survival. Regardless of the size of the component, progressive resorption of bone induced by particulate debris compromised the fixation of the femoral and acetabular components. Clearly, more time was required for the process to disrupt the larger fixation area of the larger components, indicating that higher frictional torque can be tolerated if the generation of wear debris is sufficiently limited.

The experience of surface hemiarthroplasty for avascular necrosis of the femoral head, using cemented components articulating against the host acetabulum, has clarified further the role of polyethylene wear debris in the failure of hip resurfacing [28,29]. In the absence of a polyethylene bearing, no loosening or osteolysis was observed, and the hips that required reoperation were revised for groin pain related to wear of the acetabular articular cartilage. Histologic examination of the retrieved femoral head remnants showed a thin soft tissue membrane interposed between the bone and the cement. The cement mantle was intact and the adjacent bone was viable. Contact radiographs of the slab sections showed the normal appearance of trabecular bone and no osteolytic lesions.

The femoral neck fractures seen in the first generation of hip resurfacings were, with the benefit of hindsight, due to a combination of osteolysis of the femoral neck and the surgical technique advocated at the time. Intraoperative neck notching was often a consequence of extreme valgus positioning of the implant, which was recommended to reduce the tension and shear stresses across the head-neck junction [26]. Undersizing of the implants to minimize frictional torque also resulted in notching. Trochanteric osteotomy, which was commonly used, also compromised the femoral neck if it was too extensive.

The renaissance of hip resurfacing

The renaissance of metal-on-metal articulations for total hip arthroplasty began in 1988 [30]. Weber, in collaboration with Sulzer Orthopedics (Winterthur,

Switzerland), developed the Metasul bearing, a precisely engineered, high carbon-containing, wrought Co-Cr alloy with excellent wear characteristics [31]. Large numbers of these bearings were used in Europe with good early results. The availability of a durable low-wear bearing that could be used in a large-diameter articulation enabled Heinz Wagner [32] in Germany to introduce a second-generation hip resurfacing in 1991. This system was cementless (Fig. 7). The acetabular component was a titanium alloy shell with a Metasul inlay. The thickness of the construct and the extensive macro features on its external surface made it difficult to implant. There were only four sizes available and the instruments for the preparation of the femoral head were crude. The femoral component also had two layers. The first design was screwed onto the reamed femoral head, but because of insertion difficulties, a press-fit version was developed. Only small numbers of the Wagner metal-on-metal resurfacings were used, and no long-term results are available.

In the same year in the United Kingdom, McMinn [33], in collaboration with Corin Medical (Cirencester, United Kingdom), introduced a hip resurfacing based on a cast Co-Cr alloy. The initial design was smooth surfaced and press fit on both sides (Fig. 8). The acetabular component was a modification of the Freeman finned cup. This design was associated with high incidence of early failure due to aseptic loosening of both components. The following year, the components were coated with hydroxyapatite (HA),

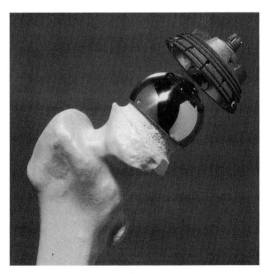

Fig. 7. The Wagner cementless metal-on-metal resurfacing. Both components consisted of two layers: a titanium alloy metal backing and a Metasul articulation. (*Courtesy of* H.C. Amstutz and P.E. Beaulé.)

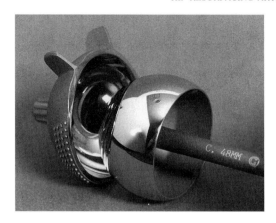

Fig. 8. The McMinn Mark I cementless metal-on-metal resurfacing system. The smooth-surfaced components were made of cast Co-Cr alloy.

but only a small number of these implants were inserted. In the same year, McMinn introduced a system in which both components were cemented. The original acetabular component was modified by removing the central peg and peripheral fins. The femoral component was not modified for cementing. This system had a high incidence of early acetabular loosening due to cement-cup debonding, which led to the introduction of a hybrid system in 1994 with a cementless HA-coated acetabulum. This implant was withdrawn in 1996, apparently because of manufacturing problems. Subsequently, two different resurfacing systems evolved. The Cormet-2000 developed by Corin Medical and the Birmingham Hip Resurfacing (Midland Medical Technologies, Birmingham, United Kingdom; now Smith & Nephew, Memphis, Tennessee). In 1996 in the United States, Amstutz introduced the Conserve Plus hybrid hip resurfacing (Wright Medical Technology, Arlington, Tennessee), with both components made of cast, heat-treated, solution-annealed Co-Cr alloy.

Contemporary hip resurfacings

By the end of 2004, most of the main implant manufacturers had introduced metal-on-metal hip resurfacing systems (Table 1). All of these systems have a number of features in common, including (1) a bearing made from high carbon-containing Co-Cr alloy, (2) cementless fixation of the acetabular component, and (3) cemented fixation of the femoral component. There are, however, important differences between these implants, particularly relating to the metallurgy and geometry of the bearing and

to aspects of the fixation of the acetabular and femoral components.

The bearing

Perhaps the most controversial issue in contemporary metal-on-metal hip resurfacing is the metallurgy of the bearing. Although all manufacturers use high carbon-containing Co-Cr alloy, the processing of the alloy differs. The alloy can be wrought or cast. If cast, the components may undergo postcasting heat treatments such as hot isostatic pressing or solution heat treatment.

The importance of postcasting heat treatments has been particularly hotly debated over the last 6 years. The annealing process results in depletion of the surface carbides, but the results from hip simulator studies demonstrate no significant difference in the wear behavior between as-cast and heat-treated alloys [34]. Until long-term clinical outcomes or reliable retrieval studies become available, it will not be possible to determine the relevance of surface carbide depletion.

Although these metallurgic differences may be important, the control of the bearing geometry is critical in determining the behavior of large-diameter metal-on-metal bearings. In particular, the radial clearance, sphericity, and surface roughness—all related to the quality of the manufacturing process—greatly influence the initial running-in wear and the steady-state wear of the bearing (see the article by Rieker et al elsewhere in this issue) [35].

Acetabular fixation

The main difference between the various contemporary resurfacing acetabular components is the surface used for bone ingrowth. Titanium vacuum plasma sprays and Co-Cr beads are currently in use. Both surfaces have been shown to have satisfactory performance when used for conventional total hip replacements; however, concern has been raised that the extreme temperature involved in the sintering process of Co-Cr beads may alter the metallurgy of the monobloc component, which in turn could have a deleterious effect on the bearing surface.

Femoral fixation

The major issue relates to the optimal cement mantle thickness and the degree of cement pressurization. The thickness of the cement mantle is determined by the diametric difference between the implant and the corresponding reamer. Systems that

Table 1
Currently marketed hip resurfacing systems

System	Introduced	Bearing		Acetabulum			Femur		
		Process	Heat treatment	Size increments (mm)	Shape	Surface	Size increments (mm)	Cement mantle (mm)	Stem
Conserve Plus (Wright Medical Technology, Arlington, Tennessee)	1996	Cast	HIP, SHT	2	Truncated hemisphere	Sintered Co-Cr beads +/− HA	2	1	+/− Load bearing
Birmingham Hip Resurfacing (Smith & Nephew, Memphis, Tennessee)	1997	Cast	None	2	Hemisphere	Co-Cr beads; cast-in + HA	4	0	Not defined
Cormet Resurfacing Hip System (Corin Medical, Cirencester, United Kingdom)	1997	Cast	HIP, SHT	2	Equatorial expansion	Ti-VPS + HA	4	0	Not defined
Durom (Zimmer, Winterthur, Switzerland)	2001	Wrought	Not applicable	2	Truncated hemisphere	Ti-VPS	2	1	Non−load bearing
ASR (Articular Surface Replacement; DePuy Orthopaedics, Warsaw, Indiana)	2003	Cast	HIP	2	Truncated hemisphere	Sintered Co-Cr beads + HA	2	0.5	Non−load bearing
ReCap (Biomet, Warsaw, Indiana)	2004	Cast	None	2	Hemisphere	Ti-VPS +/− HA	2	0.5	Not defined
Icon Hip Resurfacing (International Orthopaedics GMBH, Bromsgrove, United Kingdom)	2004	Cast	None	2	Hemisphere	Co-Cr beads; cast in + HA	4	0	Not defined

Abbreviations: HIP, hot isostatically pressed; SHT, solution heat treated; Ti-VPS, titanium vacuum plasma sprayed.

produce very thin or incomplete cement mantles and do not allow escape of cement during femoral component insertion can result in excessive penetration of cement into the cancellous bone of the femoral head. In addition, the force required to fully seat such implants can result in fracture of the femoral neck.

The role of the short stem of these implants can be for alignment alone or for alignment and force transmission. Force can be transmitted by cementation of the stem, by bony ingrowth, or by friction fit. Whether it is advantageous for the stem to transmit force remains controversial. A stem that transmits force may protect a deficient femoral head but can result in stress shielding, leading to loss of bony support in the long-term.

The Durom hip resurfacing system

In 1997, the senior authors (P.G. and P.R.), in collaboration with Sulzer Orthopedics, began the development of a new metal-on-metal hip resurfacing (Fig. 9). This development was based on the lessons learned from the history of resurfacing and metal-on-metal bearings, along with experience gained with the use of a number of implants of previous generations. The goals were to (1) produce a durable low-wear metal-on-metal articulation, (2) conserve femoral and acetabular bone stock at the time of surgery, (3) produce reliable fixation of the components, (4) avoid stress shielding of the femoral head and neck, and 5) produce sophisticated instrumentation for accurate implant sizing and safe and reproducible preparation of the femoral head. Clinical use commenced in 2001, and there have been no modifications of the implant since then.

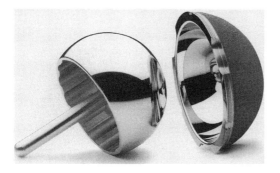

Fig. 9. The Durom hybrid hip resurfacing system designed by the senior authors (P.G. and P.R.) based on the Metasul articulation. The acetabular component has circumferential equatorial fins and a plasma-sprayed titanium coating. The femoral component is fixed with cement.

The tribology of the Durom hip resurfacing system (Zimmer, Winterthur, Switzerland) is based on the extensive experience gained with the 28-mm Metasul articulation, of which more than 250,000 have been successfully implanted since 1988. Retrieval studies and hip simulator studies have shown extremely low wear of this bearing [36,37]. The wrought, high carbon-containing Co-Cr alloy offers considerable advantages over cast Co-Cr alloys. Wrought Co-Cr is harder than cast Co-Cr (430 versus 365 HV), enhancing wear resistance [38]. The wrought alloy can also be highly polished, reducing surface roughness and enhancing lubrication.

The Metasul bearing was extensively tested in the laboratory for use in large-diameter articulations. A series of hip simulator and finite element studies were performed to optimize the diametric clearance and to investigate the resistance of the bearing to third-body wear. It was concluded that a clearance of approximately 150 μm was low enough to assure an optimum lubrication regimen but high enough to avoid the risk of clamping of the articulation due to deformation of the acetabular component under load. The bearing was found to be very resistant to the effects of abrasive particles of HA and titanium [39].

Restoration of the natural anatomy and preservation of acetabular bone stock are the essential objectives during a hip resurfacing procedure. Should revision of a resurfacing be required, it is the acetabular bone stock rather than the femoral bone stock that is critical. These objectives have been addressed with the use of 4-mm thick acetabular components available in 12 sizes with 2-mm increments. Finite element studies have shown that with a wall thickness of less than 4 mm, there is a risk that deformation under load could lead to clamping of the articulation, particularly if a low diametric clearance is used (C.B. Rieker, personal communication, 2004).

Because there is a fixed relationship between the diameter of the acetabular and femoral components, acetabular bone stock can also be compromised if the femoral component is oversized in an attempt to avoid neck notching. Prevention of this complication has been addressed by the development of a sophisticated femoral jig that allows precise implant sizing and positioning.

Primary fixation of the acetabular component is by way of a 1- to 2-mm press fit, the high surface roughness of the coating, and circumferential equatorial fins. Secondary fixation is achieved through bony ingrowth into a coating of vacuum plasma–sprayed pure titanium, a material known to have the highest biocompatibility and good potential for bone ingrowth [40].

The femoral component is fixed with acrylic cement. Finite element studies have demonstrated that a cement mantle less than 1 mm is prone to fatigue fracture under cyclic loading [41]. Although a thicker mantle reduces the risk of cement fracture, it results in increased removal of femoral head bone and could be associated with neck notching. The optimal compromise is a cement mantle of approximately 1 mm, and the instruments have been designed to achieve this. The recesses around the mouth of the femoral component facilitate controlled cement pressurization and escape, thereby allowing full seating of the component without undue force and without overpenetration of cement into the cancellous bone.

Based on the same finite element studies, the smooth, tapered stem of the Durom femoral component has been designed for alignment, not for force transmission. This design feature may reduce the risk of stress shielding of the femoral head in the long-term [41].

Early results with the Durom system

Between May 2001 and September 2003, 186 consecutive patients (200 hips) underwent a hip resurfacing using the Durom system. Operations were performed by two surgeons (P.G. and P.R.) using the posterior approach. Sixty-two percent of the patients were men and the average age was 48 years (range, 22–72 years). Sixty-three percent were Charnley category A and 27% were Charnley category B. Preoperative diagnoses included primary osteoarthritis (45%), slipped upper femoral epiphysis (20%), developmental dysplasia of the hip (18%), hip protrusio (4.5%), avascular necrosis (4%), post-traumatic arthritis (2%), and other diagnoses (6.5%). Patients were assessed clinically and radiologically at 3, 6, and 12 months and annually thereafter (Fig. 10).

No patients were lost to follow-up. There were no cases of dislocation or deep infection. There have been no failures and there are no impending failures. There were two nonfatal pulmonary embolisms. The average follow-up was 26 months (range 12–41). Respective average Charnley scores for pain, movement, and walking improved from 3, 3, and 2.5 preoperatively to 6, 5, and 5.8 postoperatively.

Two- to 4-mm interface gaps of the acetabular component were observed immediately postoperatively in nine cases. All of them showed bony filling at 6 months. One acetabular cup was fibrous fixed at 24 months. The patient is asymptomatic and maintains a high activity level. On the femoral side, there is one case of posterior neck narrowing due to bone/cup impingement. There is no evidence of acetabular or femoral migration and no evidence of focal osteolysis.

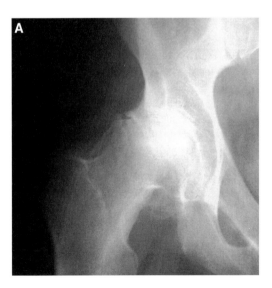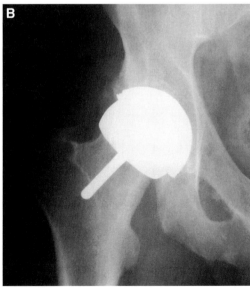

Fig. 10. (*A*) Preoperative radiograph of the right hip of a 45-year-old man with osteoarthritis secondary to slipped capital femoral epiphysis. (*B*) Radiograph taken 3 years after a Durom hip resurfacing. Components remain well fixed without any evidence of periprosthetic osteolysis.

Summary

The failure of previous generations of hip resurfacings was essentially a consequence of the use inappropriate materials, poor implant design, and inadequate instrumentation. It was not an inherent problem with the procedure itself. The early results of contemporary hip resurfacings are encouraging. The complications commonly seen in the 1970s and 1980s, such as early implant loosening and femoral neck fracture, are rare. Although early results should be regarded with caution, the present generation of metal-on-metal surface replacements potentially offers ultimate bone preservation and restoration of function in appropriately selected young patients.

Resurfacing implants demand high manufacturing standards to produce low-wear bearings consistently. Background research and better understanding of implant failure suggest that hip resurfacing technology has now developed beyond that of an experimental procedure. Concerns remain with the long-term biologic effects of the elevated metal ion levels found in all patients with metal-on-metal bearings in situ, although to date there is no evidence of any adverse clinical effect. Only long-term results and experience with this technology in the wider orthopedic community will determine whether the results will be durable or whether hip resurfacing will simply become a bone-conserving intervention before conventional total hip replacement.

Acknowledgments

The authors thank Harlan C. Amstutz and Paul E. Beaulé for providing some of the illustrations included in this article.

References

[1] Malchau H, Herberts P, Eisler T, et al. The Swedish total hip replacement register. J Bone Joint Surg Am 2002;84(Suppl 2):2–20.

[2] Amstutz HC, Grigoris P, Dorey FJ. Evolution and future of surface replacement of the hip. J Orthop Sci 1998;3:169–86.

[3] Smith-Petersen MN. Evolution of mould arthroplasty of the hip joint. J Bone Joint Surg Br 1948;30:59–75.

[4] Charnley JC. Arthroplasty of the hip: a new operation. Lancet 1961;i:1129–32.

[5] Charnley JC. Tissue reactions to polytetrafluoroethylene [letter]. Lancet 1963;ii:1379.

[6] Townley CO. Hemi and total articular replacement arthroplasty of the hip with the fixed femoral cup. Orthop Clin N Am 1982;13(4):869–94.

[7] Muller ME. Lessons of 30 years of total hip arthroplasty. Clin Orthop 1992;274:12–21.

[8] Muller ME. The benefits of metal-on-metal total hip replacements. Clin Orthop 1995;311:54–9.

[9] Gerard Y. Hip arthroplasty by matching cups. Clin Orthop 1978;134:25–35.

[10] Furuya K, Tsuchiya M, Kawachi S. Socket-cup arthroplasty. Clin Orthop 1978;134:41–4.

[11] Nishio A, Eguchi M, Kaibara N. Socket and cup surface replacement of the hip. Clin Orthop 1978;134:53–8.

[12] Tanaka S. Surface replacement of the hip joint. Clin Orthop 1978;134:75–9.

[13] Trentani C, Vaccarino F. The Paltrinieri-Trentani hip joint resurface arthroplasty. Clin Orthop 1978;134:36–40.

[14] Freeman MAR, Swanson SAV, Cameron H, et al. ICLH cemented double cup total replacement of the hip. J Bone Joint Surg Br 1978;60:137–8.

[15] Freeman MAR, Cameron HU, Brown GC. Cemented double cup arthroplasty of the hip. Clin Orthop 1978;134:45–52.

[16] Wagner H. Surface replacement arthroplasty of the hip. Clin Orthop 1978;134:102–30.

[17] Salzer M, Knahr K, Locke H, et al. Cement-free bioceramic double-cup endoprosthesis of the hip joint. Clin Orthop 1978;134:80–6.

[18] Capello WN, Ireland PH, Tramell TR, et al. Conservative total hip arthroplasty: a procedure to conserve bone stock. Part I and Part II. Clin Orthop 1978;134:59–74.

[19] Amstutz HC, Clarke IC, Cristie J, et al. Total hip articular replacement by internal eccentric shells. Clin Orthop 1977;128:261–84.

[20] Amstutz HC, Graff-Radford A, Gruen TA, et al. THARIES surface replacements. Clin Orthop 1978;134:87–101.

[21] Amstutz HC. Surface replacement arthroplasty. In: Amstutz HC, editor. Hip arthroplasty. New York: Churchill Livingstone; 1991. p. 295–333.

[22] Amstutz HC, Kabo M, Dorey FJ. Surface replacement arthroplasty: evolution of today's ingrowth-fixed design. In: Reynolds D, Freeman M, editors. Osteoarthritis in the young adult hip. Edinburgh: Churchill Livingstone; 1989. p. 251–75.

[23] Buechel FF. Resurfacing total hip replacement for avascular necrosis in young patients: durability, revision options and future technology. Presented at the 6th Annual Current Concepts in Joint Replacement Symposium. Orlando, Florida, 1990.

[24] Howie DW, Cornish BL, Vernon-Roberts B. The viability of the femoral head after resurfacing hip arthroplasty in humans. Clin Orthop 1993;291:171–84.

[25] Campbell P, Mirra J, Amstutz HC. Viability of femoral heads treated with resurfacing arthrhroplasty. J Arthroplasty 2000;15(1):120–2.

[26] Freeman MAR. Some anatomical and mechanical considerations relevant to the surface replacement of the femoral head. Clin Orthop 1978;134:19–24.

[27] Mai MT, Schmalzreid TP, Dorey FJ, et al. The contribution of frictional torque to loosening at the cement-bone interface in THARIES hip replacements. J Bone Joint Surg Am 1996;78:505–11.

[28] Amstutz HC, Grigoris P, Safran MR, et al. Precision-fit surface hemiarthroplasty for femoral head osteonecrosis: long term results. J Bone Joint Surg Br 1994;76:423–7.

[29] Grecula M, Grigoris P, Schmalzried TP, et al. Endoprostheses for osteonecrosis of the femoral head. A comparison of four models in young patients. Int Orthop 1995;19:137–43.

[30] Amstutz HC, Grigoris P. Metal-on-metal bearings in hip arthroplasty. Clin Orthop 1996;329:S11–34.

[31] Weber BG. Experience with the Metasul total hip bearing system. Clin Orthop 1996;329S:S69–77.

[32] Wagner M, Wagner H. Preliminary results of uncemented metal-on-metal stemmed and resurfacing hip replacement arthroplasty. Clin Orthop 1996;329:S78–88.

[33] McMinn D, Treacy R, Lin K, et al. Metal-on-metal surface replacement of the hip. Clin Orthop 1996;329:S89–98.

[34] Bowsher JG, Nevelos J, Pickard J, et al. Do heat treatments influence the wear of large metal-on-metal hip joints? An in vitro study under normal and adverse conditions. Presented at the 49th Annual Meeting of the Orthopaedic Research Society. New Orleans, Louisiana. February 2003.

[35] Chan FW, Bobyn JD, Medley JB, et al. Wear and lubrication of metal-on-metal hip implants. Clin Orthop 1999;369:10–24.

[36] Sieber HP, Rieker CB, Kottig P. Analysis of 118 second generation metal-on-metal retrieved hip implants. J Bone Joint Surg Br 1999;81:46–50.

[37] Rieker CB, Kottig P. In-vivo tribological performance of 231 metal-on-metal hip articulations. Hip Int 2002;12:73–6.

[38] Archard JF. Contact and rubbing of flat surfaces. J Appl Phys 1953;24:981–8.

[39] Rieker CB, Konrad R, Schon R, et al. Effect of third body abrasive wear particles on the wear behaviour of modern metal-on-metal articulations. Transactions of the 2001 Meeting of the European Society for Biomaterials.

[40] Wilke A, Knoell P, Frank H, et al. Osteointegration of vacuum-plasma-sprayed (VPS) titanium implants with/without hydroxyapatite coating. Presented at the 7th World Biomaterial Congress. Sydney, Australia, May 2004.

[41] Soulhat J, Hertig D, Ploeg H, et al. Finite element analysis of a cemented hip resurfacing. J Bone Joint Surg Br 2003;85(Suppl I):7.

ELSEVIER
SAUNDERS

Orthop Clin N Am 36 (2005) 135 – 142

ORTHOPEDIC
CLINICS
OF NORTH AMERICA

Influence of the Clearance on In-Vitro Tribology of Large Diameter Metal-on-Metal Articulations Pertaining to Resurfacing Hip Implants

Claude B. Rieker, PhD[a],*, Rolf Schön[a], Reto Konrad[a], Gernot Liebentritt[a], Patric Gnepf[a], Ming Shen[a], Paul Roberts, MA(Oxon), MB, FRCS[b], Peter Grigoris, FRCS, FACS[c,d]

[a]Tribology–113 955, Zimmer Europe GmbH, Sulzer Allee 8, CH 8404 Winterthur, Switzerland
[b]Department of Orthopaedics and Trauma, Royal Gwent Hospital, Cardiff Road, Newport NP9 2UB, Wales, UK
[c]2nd Orthopaedic Department, University of Athens, Ag. Olga Hospital, 142 33 N. Ionia, Athens, Greece
[d]Department of Medical Engineering, School of Engineering, Design, and Technology, University of Bradford, Richmond Road, Bradford, West Yorkshire BD7 1DP, UK

Aseptic loosening [1] due to osteolysis induced by polyethylene wear debris [2] is known as the most common cause of long-term failure in total hip joint prostheses. An increasing number of publications have reported direct correlations between the amount of polyethylene wear and the incidence of aseptic loosening [3] or between the amount of polyethylene wear and the incidence of revisions [4]. Alternative surface articulations such as metal-on-metal, alumina-on-alumina, or highly cross-linked polyethylenes have been developed to reduce this phenomenon. Metal-on-metal articulations have demonstrated a significant decrease in the amount of wear in vitro [5] and in vivo [6]. Good clinical results have also been reported from second-generation metal-on-metal articulations (head diameter, 28 or 32 mm) since the late 1980s [7–9]. Moreover, the metal ion concentrations measured in serum or blood of patients having the second-generation metal-on-metal articulations have been low (range, 0.5–2 μg/L) [10,11].

These findings clearly suggest that the wear of modern metal-on-metal articulations is low. To date, a causal link has never been demonstrated between cancer risks or any other long-term clinical issues and metal ions in patients with metal-on-metal implants [12,13]. Nevertheless, a better understanding of the lubrication modes in metal-on-metal articulations will allow for better control of their wear behavior and potentially reduce metal ion levels further. It may also provide insights for the development of new designs that allow the introduction of improved metal-on-metal resurfacing hip implants.

The form of lubrication occurring in a total hip prosthesis can be expressed by the film thickness ratio (lambda coefficient) as defined in the equation

$$\text{Lambda coefficient} = \frac{h_c}{\sqrt{(Rq_{Head})^2 + (Rq_{Cup})^2}} \quad (1)$$

where h_c is the central film thickness, Rq_{Head} is the root mean square roughness of the head, and Rq_{Cup} is the root mean square roughness of the cup [14]. The value of the lambda coefficient provides an indication of the lubrication mode. With a lambda coefficient greater than 3, there is a complete fluid film, with negligible contact between the head and the cup.

Benefits and funds were received from Zimmer GmbH in partial or total support of the research material described in this article.

* Corresponding author.
E-mail address: claude.rieker@zimmer.com
(C.B. Rieker).

When the lambda coefficient is less than 3, the lubrication may involve mixed films, some elasto-hydrodynamic lubrication film, or boundary lubrication film. In such cases, some contacts will take place between the head and the cup and generate some amount of wear.

Recently published works [15,16] have shown that large diameter metal-on-metal articulations with smaller clearances offer the possibility of reaching a complete fluid film lubrication (lambda coefficient >3), which should help minimize the amount of wear. From a clinical perspective, the enhanced lubrication in a large diameter metal-on-metal articulation permits the use of a large femoral head in a total hip replacement that offers improved range of motion and stability. Such large diameter articulations also enable the use of resurfacing arthroplasties, with additional advantages of more physiologic load transmission and an increased number of options for surgical intervention in the case of a clinical failure [17,18].

This article describes the study in which the authors used a hip joint simulator to investigate the influence of clearance and diameter on wear of large diameter metal-on-metal hip-resurfacing implant prototypes made of high-carbon, wrought-forged, cobalt-chrome alloy. The wear amounts, in terms of linear wear rate, were measured periodically during the wear test. After the test, representative wear surfaces were characterized. The post-test wear analysis was performed using wear measurements and typical wear surface characteristics. Based on the results, the functional dependency of wear on the diameter and the clearance was examined. The authors also address the implications of the wear results regarding potential lubrication modes operating in large diameter metal-on-metal articulations.

Methods

All of the tested components were manufactured from a high carbon (0.20%– 0.25% carbon),

Table 1
Specimens tested with varying diameter and clearance

Diameter (mm)	Diametrical clearance (μm)	No. of components tested
38	96.9 ± 5.4	4
38	278.4 ± 25.4	4
50	144.8 ± 5.4	4
50	263.2 ± 26.8	4
54	65.6 ± 15.4	6
56	237.9 ± 13.6	4

Table 2
Test conditions used as specified in International Standards Organization standard 14242-1

Properties	Value
Flexion/extension	25°/18°
Abduction/adduction	7°/4°
Internal/external rotation	10°/2°
Maximum load (double peak)	3000 N
Temperature	37°C
Frequency	1.0 Hz
No. of cycles	5 million

wrought-forged, cobalt-chrome alloy (PROTASUL-21WF, Zimmer GmbH, Winterthur, Switzerland) in accordance with the International Standards Organization standard 5832-11. Six combinations of diameters and clearances were investigated in this study (Table 1). These combinations were chosen to cover sufficiently wide ranges of diameter and clearance such that the results could be useful in establishing a baseline of how large diameter metal-on-metal articulations behave while keeping the values close to what could readily be manufactured on a large scale.

The metal-on-metal components were tested on a hip simulator (Boston Hip Simulator, AMTI, Watertown, Massachusetts) that was operated hydraulically with the kinematics specified in Table 2 (International Standards Organization standard 14242-1), mimicking walking gait. The components were lubricated with a stabilized mixture of Ringer's solution consisting of 33% newborn calf serum (2-02F90, BioConcept, Allschwil, Switzerland) buffered to a pH of 7.2. The proteins and salts of this lubricant mimicked those of healthy human synovial fluid [5]. The lubricant was filtered with a 0.2-μm filter before testing. During the test, the lubricant temperature was maintained at 37°C ± 2°C, and the lubricant was replaced after every 0.5 million cycles.

The wear of the components was measured by means of a coordinate measuring machine (CMM5, SIP, Geneva, Switzerland), with a measurement resolution of less than 1 μm. The measurements were made every 5° on 12 concentric circles and at the poles of the components (1297 measurements for the heads and 1153 for the cups). The surface dimensions of the head and the cup were measured with the coordinate measuring machine before each experiment. These measurements were used to establish reference geometries and were compared with the measurements made every 0.5 or 1.0 million cycles thereafter. The amount of wear, defined by the

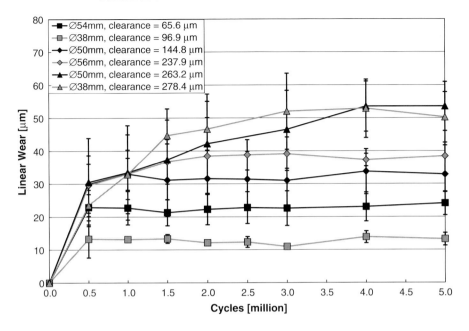

Fig. 1. Linear wear as a function of the number of cycles.

maximum deviation from the reference geometry, was calculated by comparing the measurements made (after a given number of cycles) with the reference geometries. Due to the uncertainties associated with repositioning the components on the coordinate measuring machine and with random occurrence of permanent organic films deposited on the articulating surface of the components, the precision of the wear measurements was estimated to be about ± 2 μm.

At the end of the wear tests, two femoral heads were examined using scanning electronic microscopy (JSM-840, JEOL, Tokyo, Japan). The two heads were selected from 50-mm diameter couples, representing the midrange diameter and covering sufficiently large clearance differences. Surface features inside the loaded zones were observed and compared with those reported in a 28-mm diameter design [6]. Surface roughness was analyzed for the two femoral heads using a stylus surface analyzer (Perthometer PRK, Mahr-Perthometer, Göttingen, Germany) with the following parameters: measurement length, 1.50 mm; cut-off length, 0.25 mm. The two heads were selected from the two low-clearance cases (see Table 1): 38-mm diameter with a 96.9-μm clearance and 54-mm diameter with a 65.6-μm clearance. For each femoral head, surface roughness was measured in two areas: at the pole (loaded zone) and near the equator (unloaded zone). A minimum of 10 traces was collected in each of the two areas. From

those traces, the following roughness parameters were calculated:

$$R_a = \frac{1}{l} \int_0^l |Z(x)| dx \qquad (2)$$

$$R_{sk} = \frac{1}{l(Rq)^3} \int_0^l |Z^3(x)| dx \qquad (3)$$

where R_a is the average roughness, R_{sk} is the skewness, l is measurement length, Z is the height of the surface, and Rq is the root mean square roughness of the component.

Table 3
Wear amounts and durations in the running-in periods

Diameter (mm)	Diametrical clearance (μm)	Linear running-in wear (μm)	No. of cycles for the running-in period (millions)
38	96.9 ± 5.4	13.3	0.5
38	278.4 ± 25.4	52.0	3
50	144.8 ± 5.4	33.0	1
50	263.2 ± 26.8	53.5	4
54	65.6 ± 15.4	22.9	0.5
56	237.9 ± 13.6	38.5	2

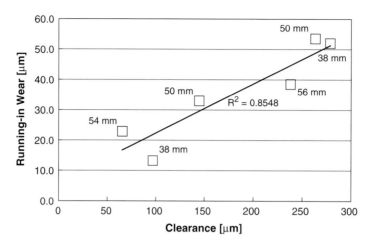

Fig. 2. Influence of the clearance on the amount of linear running-in wear.

Average roughness and skewness reflect the symmetry in the surface roughness. Surfaces with a positive skewness have peaks protruding above the surface, whereas surfaces with a negative skewness have valleys in a plateau.

Results

Wear

Fig. 1 shows the wear curves of the six tested systems. A common behavior was displayed in all of the wear tests: a well-defined running-in period followed by a period in which there was no increase in the measured amount of wear (if there was any systematic linear wear after the running-in period, it was below the resolution of the coordinate measuring machine). The characteristics of the running-in wear of the six wear curves are listed in Table 3. The amounts of linear wear associated with the running-in wear varied from 13.3 μm to 53.5 μm. The durations of the running-in wear ranged from 0.5 to 4.0 million cycles. These characteristics were further analyzed graphically as a function of the respective clearance values.

Fig. 2 displays the influence of clearance on the amount of linear wear in the running-in period. A linear regression between the clearance and the amount of running-in wear showed that a correlation existed ($R^2 = 0.86$, $P = 0.01$). Specifically, the lower the clearance within the tested range, the lower the

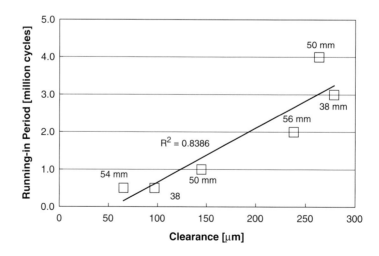

Fig. 3. Influence of the clearance on the number of cycles of the running-in period.

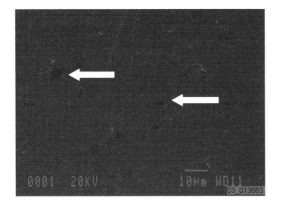

Fig. 4. Pole (loaded zone) of a head after 5 million cycles.

Table 4
Measured surface roughness parameters of two femoral heads after testing

Femoral head	Average roughness	Skewness
Unloaded	0.021 ± 0.006 µm	0.52 ± 0.63
Loaded	0.010 ± 0.004 µm	-0.40 ± 2.76

amount of measured running-in wear. The nominal diameter of the bearing did not have any apparent influence on this behavior. Fig. 3 exhibits the influence of clearance on the number of cycles of the running-in period. A linear regression between the clearance and the number of cycles of the running-in period showed that a correlation also existed ($R^2 = 0.84$, $P = 0.01$). Specifically, the lower the clearance within the tested range, the fewer cycles in the running-in period. Similar to the functional dependence exhibited in the amount of linear wear, the nominal diameter of the bearing did not have any apparent influence on this behavior.

Wear surface

A typical example of femoral head surfaces around the pole (loaded zone) after 5 million cycles is shown in Fig. 4. In addition, a typical surface in the

unloaded zones is shown in Fig. 5. These two figures exhibit the following features:

- Carbides (arrows) approximately 5 µm in diameter were embedded in the metallic matrix.
- The wear surface in the loaded zone was smooth, with only a small number of multidirectional scratches detectable. In contrast, some shallow grooves were present in the unloaded zones, which were presumed to be remnants from the machining/polishing process.

Roughness

Table 4 lists the roughness parameters measured from two femoral components after 5 million cycles. Comparing the unloaded zone to the loaded zone, a decrease in the average roughness from 0.021 µm to 0.010 µm was observed (ie, the loaded zone had a smoother wear surface after the test). A Student t test at 95% confidence level with equal variances showed the decrease was statistically significant ($P < 0.01$). Meanwhile, the skewness was mostly positive in the unloaded zone but had some negative values in the loaded zone, presumably due to the presence of scratches. The average skewness decreased from 0.52 in the unloaded zones to -0.40 in the loaded zones.

Discussion

According to the authors' knowledge, the present investigation is the first study of its kind to experimentally explore the influences of the nominal bearing diameter and diametral clearance on the wear behavior of large metal-on-metal articulations. The influence of clearance on the wear behavior of smaller metal-on-metal articulations (28-mm diameter) was reported by Chan et al [19] in a hip simulator study of 22 components. Their results showed that the wear amount increased with increasing diametral clearance from 16 bearings with diametral clearances between 30 µm and 110 µm and with roughness values of 5 to 10 nm. A second-order polynomial relationship ($R^2 = 0.65$, $P = 0.001$) between the

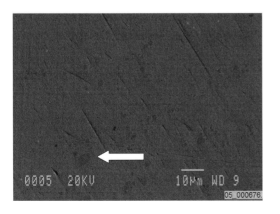

Fig. 5. Unloaded zone of a head after 5 million cycles.

total wear volume and the diametral clearance was reported [19]. By plotting the tabulated running-in wear data against the clearance of the same group of 16 bearings [19], a slightly better correlation ($R^2 = 0.72$) could be obtained with a second-order polynomial relationship. These second-order polynomial relationships suggested that wear continued to occur after the running-in period in those 28-mm bearings, although at a much-reduced rate. The reduction in wear after running-in suggested that the lubrication mode had improved and some level of fluid film lubrication, presumably a mixed film lubrication mode, might be present. In contrast, the results of the present study show that a linear relationship existed ($R^2 = 0.86$) between the running-in wear and the diametral clearance. Meanwhile, the amounts of linear wear after the running-in period, if any, were too small to detect. Such characteristics suggest that these large diameter metal-on-metal articulations had a different wear behavior compared with the 28-mm bearings. For these large diameter metal-on-metal articulations, the diametral clearance affected the wear behaviors only in the running-in period. After the running-in period, the negligible wear phenomena appeared to be benefited by a much improved lubrication mode in which a separation between the femoral head and the acetabular cup by a fluid film might have existed.

Smith et al [15] observed a similar wear benefit in 36-mm diameter metal-on-metal articulations from an in vitro wear test. Significantly lower steady-state wear rates after the running-in period existed in the 36-mm bearings compared with the 28-mm bearings under the same test conditions. In addition, theoretic analyses by Udofia and Jin [16] and Chan et al [20] indicated that large metal-on-metal articulations had a higher propensity to generate continuous fluid films separating the two mating parts. These findings supported the nearly negligible wear phenomena observed after the running-in period in this study.

The findings of the wear surface analysis, performed after the test, were in agreement with the wear data. The scanning electron microscopy observations in Figs. 4 and 5 depicted smoother wear surfaces accompanied by a few multidirectional scratches in the loaded zones compared with the unloaded zone. An approximately 50% decrease in the average roughness in the loaded zone (see Table 4) compared with the value in the unloaded zone confirmed that the wear surfaces became smoother after the test. The scratches present in the loaded zone did not cause an increase in the average roughness. The features of the smoother wear surfaces were consistent with the previously reported self-polishing

effects during the running-in phase [21,22]. Presumably, the surface roughness peaks protruding above the surface were worn off during the running-in period [23]. Accordingly, one would expect a decrease in the skewness value. The formation of grooves on the surface, as evidenced by the presence of scratches, would further decrease the skewness value. Hence, negative skewness values found in the loaded zones after the test were reasonable as a result of the combined effects of the two processes: the removal of surface roughness peaks and the formation of grooves. The observed changes in the surface roughness and the skewness after the test implied that a shift in the lubrication mode took place, presumably as the wear process transitioned from the running-in period to steady-state wear.

Assuming a 50% reduction in the average roughness of the head (as observed in this study) and of the cup, the lambda coefficient would be doubled according to Eq. 1. Although no roughness measurements were performed with the cup components in the present study, their wear surfaces would also have become smoother by the self-polishing wear process. The combined self-polishing effects in the two mating components would decrease the denominator in Eq. 1, thus raising the lambda coefficient. Meanwhile, the wear process during the running-in period would also change the contact curvatures in the head and the cup. Such changes would result in an increase in the "combined" contact radius, which in turn would promote a thicker fluid film in the contact [15,19]; that is, the numerator in Eq. 1 would increase as a result of the running-in wear. Combining an increase in the film thickness term with decreases in the surface roughness terms in Eq. 1, a net increase in the lambda coefficient is realized, bringing the lubrication mode closer toward full-film lubrication. The nearly negligible wear observed after the running-in period suggested a high probability for the operating lubrication mode to be in full-film lubrication.

The wear results of all of the head–cup pairs in the present study demonstrated similarly that wear became negligible after the running-in period, despite the initial diameters or initial clearances. That is, the initial clearance affected the amount of linear running-in wear and the number of cycles of the running-in period. These observations led to the following two conclusions:

1. Within the system described in the present investigation, a head diameter of 38 mm was large enough to promote lubrication that resulted in an extremely low (almost nil) steady-state wear after the running-in period.

2. The clearance should be as small as possible within a range that avoids a clamping phenomenon. The two articulating surfaces—head and cup—adapted to each other during the running-in period. Thus, additional cycles and more wear were required in larger clearance cases before a steady-state condition could be reached.

There are limitations to these conclusions. The first conclusion might not be applicable for other types of large metal-on-metal articulations, especially for those manufactured with rougher surfaces. A large diameter promotes the formation of a thicker fluid film, but rougher surfaces disrupt the film. As the lambda coefficient dictates, a rough surface would bring the lubrication mode away from a continuous fluid film condition. Typical cast cobalt-chrome alloys tend to have larger carbide particles in the raw material compared with the wrought-forged cobalt-chrome alloy employed in the present study. Thus, care needs to be taken to assure that the surface roughness of the articulating surfaces is at least similar to or smaller than the values employed in this study.

With regard to the second conclusion, due to the deformation in the acetabular cup under load, a minimum clearance will be mandatory to avoid equatorial clamping that may lead to a high frictional torque and, thus, potentially cause loosening of the acetabular component [24]. It is extremely difficult, however, to assess the minimum clearance requirement because various factors influence the in vivo deformation of the articulation (eg, body weight of the patient, activities of the patient, quality of the bone, amount of press-fit, relative position of the implants, design of the components, and so forth).

Finally, the results suggest that a complete fluid film lubrication is possible in vitro with this particular type of hip resurfacing prototype made of wrought-forged, cobalt-chrome alloy, although the experimental conditions were somewhat idealized; that is the same walking motions were repeated without any interruption for 0.5 or 1 million cycles. The actual in vivo conditions would differ considerably from the in vitro situations, with the juxtaposition of different activities of daily living and stop-and-go motions making the continuous fluid film lubrication impossible to maintain all the time. Thus, the mixed lubrication could be a prevailing lubrication mode in the in vivo situation. Nevertheless, because only a few cycles are needed to generate continuous fluid film lubrication [14], the full-film lubrication mode may still be an operating lubrication mode in vivo for large metal-on-metal articulations.

Summary

This study showed that clearance was a key factor in controlling the running-in wear behavior in large metal-on-metal articulations. A small clearance minimized the amount of wear during the running-in period, which would translate to a reduction in the metallic burden endured in patients. Moreover, under the experimental conditions of this study, a lubrication mode consisting of a continuous fluid film was highly likely to exist for metal-on-metal articulations with diameters equal to or larger than 38 mm. Therefore, large diameter metal-on-metal articulations is a promising concept for total hip arthroplasty.

References

[1] Malchau H, Herberts P, Eisler T, et al. The Swedish total hip replacement register. J Bone and Joint Surg Am 2002;84(Suppl 2):2–20.

[2] Harris WH. Wear and periprosthetic osteolysis. Clin Orthop 2001;393:66–70.

[3] Oparaugo PC, Clarke IC, Malchau H, et al. Correlation of wear debris-induced osteolysis and revision with volumetric wear-rates of polyethylene—a survey of 8 reports in the literature. Acta Orthop Scand 2001;72: 22–8.

[4] Sochard DH. Relationship of acetabular wear to osteolysis and loosening in total hip arthroplasty. Clin Orthop 1999;363:135–50.

[5] Streicher RM, Semlitsch M, Schön R, et al. Metal-on-metal articulation for artificial hip joints: laboratory study and clinical results. Proc Instn Mech Engrs 1996;210:223–32.

[6] Sieber HP, Rieker CB, Koettig P. Analysis of 118 second-generation metal-on-metal retrieved hip implants. J Bone and Joint Surg Br 1999;81: 46–50.

[7] Wagner M, Wagner H. Medium-term results of a modern metal-on-metal system in total hip. Clin Orthop 2000;379:123–33.

[8] Delaunay C. Metasul articulation survey in primary total hip arthroplasty consecutive series of 100 cementless Alloclassic-Metasul hips. In: Rieker C, Oberholzer S, Wyss U, editors. World tribology forum in arthroplasty. Berne, Switzerland: Hans Huber; 2001. p. 189–96.

[9] Doerig MF, Kratter R, Ritzler T, et al. Ceramic-on-polyethylene versus metal-on-metal: a clinical and radiological follow up study, five to ten years after implantation. In: Rieker C, Oberholzer S, Wyss U, editors. World tribology forum in arthroplasty. Berne, Switzerland: Hans Huber; 2001. p. 197–226.

[10] Brodner W, Bitzan P, Meisinger V, et al. Serum cobalt levels after metal-on-metal total hip arthroplasty. J Bone and Joint Surg Am 2003;85:2168–73.

[11] Savarino L, Granchi D, Ciapetti G, et al. Ion release in patients with metal-on-metal hip bearings in TJR: a comparison with metal-on-polyethylene bearings. J Biomed Mater Res 2002;63:467–74.

[12] Visuri T. Does metal-on-metal THP have influence on cancer? In: Rieker C, Oberholzer S, Wyss U, editors. World tribology forum in arthroplasty. Berne, Switzerland: Hans Huber; 2001. p. 181–7.

[13] MacDonald SJ. Metal-on-metal total hip arthroplasty: the concerns. Clin Orthop 2004;429:86–93.

[14] Medley JB, Bobyn JD, Krygier JJ, et al. Elasto-hydrodynamic lubrication and wear of metal-on-metal hip implant. In: Rieker C, Oberholzer S, Wyss U, editors. World tribology forum in arthroplasty. Berne, Switzerland: Hans Huber; 2001. p. 125–36.

[15] Smith SL, Dowson D, Goldsmith AAJ. The effect of femoral head diameter upon lubrication and wear of metal-on-metal total hip replacements. Proc Instn Mech Engrs 2001;215:161–70.

[16] Udofia IJ, Jin ZM. Elastohydrodynamic lubrication analysis of metal-on-metal hip-resurfacing prostheses. J Biomech 2003;36:537–44.

[17] McMinn D, Treacy R, Lin K, et al. Metal-on-metal surface replacement of the hip—experience with the McMinn prosthesis. Clin Orthop 1996;329S:89–98.

[18] Amstutz HC, Grigoris P, Dorey FJ. Evolution and future of surface replacement of the hip. J Orthop Sci 1998;3:169–86.

[19] Chan FW, Bobyn JD, Medley JB, et al. Wear and lubrication of metal-on-metal hip implants. Clin Orthop 1999;369:11–24.

[20] Chan FW, Medley JB, Bobyn JD, et al. Numerical analysis of time-varying, fluid film thickness in metal-metal hip implants in simulator tests. In: Jacobs JJ, Craig TL, editors. Alternative articulation surfaces in total joint replacement. West Conshohocken (PA): ASTM; 1998. p. 111–28.

[21] Park SH, McKellop H, Lu B, et al. Wear morphology of metal-metal implants: hip simulator tests compared with clinical retrievals. In: Jacobs JJ, Craig TL, editors. Alternative articulation surfaces in total joint replacement. West Conshohocken (PA): ASTM; 1998. p. 129–43.

[22] Goldsmith AAJ, Dowson D, Issac GH, et al. Wear morphology of metal-metal implants: hip simulator tests compared with clinical retrievals. Proc Instn Mech Engrs 2000;214:39–47.

[23] Williams JA. Engineering tribology. Oxford, UK: Oxford Science Publications; 1994.

[24] Walker PS, Gold BL. The tribology (friction, lubrication and wear) of all-metal artificial hip joints. Wear 1971;17:285–99.

ELSEVIER
SAUNDERS

Orthop Clin N Am 36 (2005) 143 – 162

ORTHOPEDIC
CLINICS
OF NORTH AMERICA

Current Concepts of Metal-on-Metal Hip Resurfacing

Ian C. Clarke, PhD[a,*], Thomas Donaldson, MD[b], John G. Bowsher, PhD[a],
Sam Nasser, MD, PhD[c,d], Tomoki Takahashi, MD[e]

[a]Orthopedic Research Center, 11406 Loma Linda Drive #606, Loma Linda University Medical Center,
Loma Linda, CA 92354, USA
[b]Department of Orthopedics, Loma Linda University Medical Center, 11406 Loma Linda Drive #606,
Loma Linda, CA 92354, USA
[c]Department of Orthopedics, School of Medicine, Wayne State University, Detroit, MI, USA
[d]Department of Biomedical Engineering, College of Engineering, Wayne State University, Detroit, MI, USA
[e]Department of Orthopaedic Surgery, Kumamoto University of Medicine, Yamamuro 6-8-1, Kumamoto City, 860-8518,
Kumamoto Prefecture, Japan

Femoral resurfacing has spanned four technologic phases over an 80-year history (Table 1) [1–3]. The 1920s brought in the pioneering use of various materials as press-fit, interpositional, and hemiarthroplasty resurfacing concepts (see the article by Grigoris et al elsewhere in this issue). Advances in the 1950 to 1960 era ushered in attempts to resurface femoral and acetabular cartilages. The first series of metal-on-metal (MOM) total hip replacements (THRs) entailed 26 operations conducted between 1956 and 1960 [4]. The initial ball diameter was approximately 32 mm, followed by 42 mm in 1960; a 35 mm diameter was added in 1966. In those pioneering attempts, approximately 30% to 40% were revised mainly due to impingement, with observations of varying amounts of sludge containing many metal particles [5]. In 1967, MOM press-fit resurfacing with 43-mm shells was initiated but abandoned in favor of THR with polyethylene cups in 1968. Thus, the "big-ball" MOM paradigm began 44 years ago with the 42-mm diameter THR and 37 years ago with resurfacing.

The advent of the cemented THR in the 1960s ushered in a completely new paradigm. Charnley

et al [6] introduced the concept of a uniquely small ball (22.25 mm) in a cemented ultra-high molecular weight polyethylene (UHMWPE) cup. From clinical and revision observations of this original polytetrafluoroethylene series, these investigators noted that progressively downsizing the femoral ball (41.5 to 22.25 mm) led to noticeably less wear in vivo, even with the now notorious polytetrafluoroethylene material (Fig. 1) [7]. The "small-ball" wear paradigm, however, was lost in time with the progression of larger ball development in the United States due to balancing dislocation risks against wear issues [7,8]. The resurfacing concepts launched in the 1970s and 1980s (see Table 1) used even larger diameter balls (see Fig. 1) and introduced the thin-walled UHMWPE cup. In 1982, Clarke [1] reviewed the status of this third era of resurfacing designs. It is unfortunate that resurfacing's big-ball paradigm in this era produced significant UHMWPE wear debris with concomitantly higher revision rates (see the article by Grigoris et al elsewhere in this issue). Over time, the UHMWPE cups have again restricted the surgeons' choices to the original small-ball paradigm of Charnley.

In the late 1980s, the second-generation MOM bearing for THR was launched using the 28-mm ball (see Table 1). Surgeons quickly appreciated that the low-wear characteristics of MOM bearings permitted use of the more desirable big-ball concept, which provided added stability and range of motion. Thus,

---

* Corresponding author.
E-mail address: iclarke@som.llu.edu (I.C. Clarke).

0030-5898/05/$ – see front matter © 2005 Elsevier Inc. All rights reserved.
doi:10.1016/j.ocl.2005.02.007

orthopedic.theclinics.com

Table 1
Four developmental phases of materials technology used for resurfacing the human hip

Surgery (y)	Author	Femoral shell	Acetabular cup
1923	Smith-Petersen	Press-fit glass	NA
1938	**Smith-Petersen**	Press-fit **CoCr**	NA
1951	Charnley	Press-fit PTFE	Press-fit PTFE
1953	**Haboush**	**Cement-CoCr**	**Cement-CoCr**
1960	Townley	CoCr	Polyurethane
1961	**McKee**	**THR-cement**	**Cement-CoCr**
1963	Charnley	Cemented THR	Cement PE
1967	Mueller	Press-fit CoCr	Press-fit CoCr
1967	Weber	THR-cement	Cement-CoCr
1970	**Gerard**	**Cement-CoCr**	**Cement-CoCr**
1970	Townley	Press-fit CoCr	Cement-PE
1971	Furuya	Stainless steel	Cement-PE
1971	Paltrinieri	Cement-CoCr	Cement-PE
1972	Freeman	Cement-CoCr	Cement-PE
1973	Townley	Cement-CoCr	Cement-PE
1975	Amstutz	Cement-CoCr	Cement-PE
1977	Townley	Cement-CoCr	Cement-PE
1982	Wagner	Cement-CoCr	Cement-PE
1982	Wagner	Cement-Al_2O_3	Cement-PE
1982	Amstutz	Cement-CoCr	Porous MB-PE
1988	Amstutz	Porous-CoCr	Porous MB-PE
1988	**Weber**	**THR (Metasul)**	**1pc cement PE/CoCr**
1991	**Dorr**	**THR (Metasul)**	**1pc cement PE/CoCr**
1991	McMinn	Cement-CoCr	Cement-CoCr
1994	McMinn	Cement-CoCr (stem)	Porous/HA-CoCr
1994	Amstutz	Porous-CoCr	Porous MB-PE
1995	**FDA-approved**	**Cement-CoCr (stem)**	**None (hemiarthroplasty)**
1996	Amstutz	Cement-CoCr (stem)	Porous-CoCr
1997	McMinn	Cement-CoCr (stem)	Porous/HA-CoCr
1999	**FDA-approved**	**28mm THR (Metasul)**	**Modular, CoCr PE-sandwich cup**
2000	**Biomet**	**M2a**	**MOM 28, 32 mm**
2001	Grigoris	Cement-CoCr (stem)	Plasma-spray/Ti-CoCr
2001	**Anastasios**	**Porous/HA-CoCr**	**Porous/HA-CoCr**
2001	**Biomet**	**M2a**	**MOM 38 mm**
2001	**Wright Medical Tech**	**LINEAGE THR**	**MOM 28, 32 mm**
2002	**Wright Medical Tech**	**BFH THR**	**MOM 36–56 mm**
2003	**Biomet**	**Magnum THR**	**MOM 38–60 mm dia.**

Advent of CoCr implant innovations and milestone clinical studies are shown in bold. Metasul (Zimmer/CenterPulse Inc); BFH (Wright Medical Inc); LINEAGE (Wright Medical Inc); Magnum (Biomet Inc).
Abbreviations: CoCr, cobalt-chromium; dia., diameter; FDA, Food and Drug Administration; HA, hydroxyapatite; MB, metal-backed; MOM, metal-on-metal; NA, not available; PE, polyethylene; PTFE, polytetrafluoroethylene; THR, total hip replacement.
Data from Refs. [1–3].

the use of MOM reversed Charnley's small-ball paradigm. The tremendous impact of the big-ball paradigm can be visualized by the scaling of ball diameters (see Fig. 1). Compared with the 28-mm THR size, the 38- and 54-mm resurfacing added 30% to 90% additional range of motion (approximately 1° range of motion

added per 1 mm of diameter). The high-strength cobalt-chromium (CoCr) alloy also facilitated the design of the "thin" acetabular cup combined with the now-standard, porous-coating layer for fixation. Twenty-two years later [1], the authors have a second opportunity to analyze the direction of contemporary resurfacing

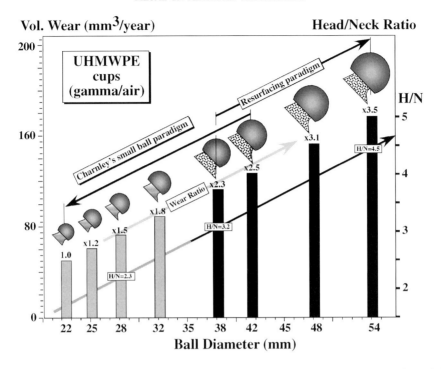

Fig. 1. Wear rates of UHMWPE cups indicated with 1.8-fold wear increase over the 22 to 32 mm range of THR ball sizes [7]. Prior clinical experience with polytetrafluoroethylene cups also showed this paradigm [6] and led to a downsizing in femoral balls from 41.5 mm to 22.25 mm, ie, Charnley's 'small ball' paradigm produced the least UHMWPE wear. Dramatic size of scale is evident between the range of THR balls (22–32 mm) and femoral resurfacing shells (38–54 mm). Also shown are the nominal head/neck ratios (H/N; 12 mm diameter neck assumed) increasing from 2.3 with 28 mm ball to 4.5 with 54 mm ball, thereby conferring greater range of motion and stability with the 'large ball' paradigm.

concepts. This review examines femoral fixation, bone remodeling, and wear studies of MOM implants and provides a brief overview of the latest outcome and retrieval data and how these data integrate with the in vitro wear studies.

Resurfacing concerns in the 1980s

The search for the optimal resurfacing concept has weathered many challenges (Table 2). The most dramatic challenge of the 1980 to 1990 era was the

Table 2
Summary of potential risks circa 1982 related to hip resurfacing implants

Parameter	Feature	Risk circa 1982
Over-reaming femur	Neck notching	Stress riser, fracture
Over-reaming acetabulum	Inadequate support	Loosening of cemented cup
Metal-backed, PE-liner	Noncemented	Unknown
Cement technique	Shell fixation	Loosening (necrosis?)
Incomplete coverage of reamed head	Stress riser	Neck fracture
Impingement	Neck narrowing?	Not a clinical problem
Rigid CoCr shells	Abnormal stresses	Detrimental remodeling?
Femoral stem	Guide and stabilizer	Unknown
High frictional torque	Loosening	Not a clinical problem
UHMWPE debris	Osteolysis	Implant loosening

Abbreviation: PE, polyethylene.
Data from Clarke IC. Symposium on surface replacement arthroplasty of the hip. Biomechanics: mutifactorial design choices—an essential compromise? Orthop Clin N Am 1982;13(4):681–707; and Clarke IC. Wear-screening and joint simulation studies vs materials selection and prosthesis design. Crc Crit Rev Biomed Eng 1982;8(1):29–91.

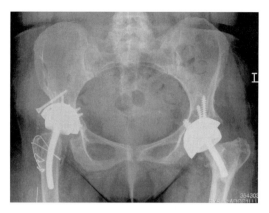

Fig. 2. A low-activity, female patient with multiple hip operations with bilateral TARA implants (UHMWPE liners) followed nearly 20 years. Now at age 40 years, reoperation of right hip (Loma Linda University Medical Center, January 2005) confirmed there was no bone inside the femoral shell. The curved TARA stem was left well fixed inside the remaining stump of proximal neck. In contrast, the left hip showed considerable sclerosis around a much shorter stem, with bone bridging to medial and lateral cortices. These features are shown schematically for emphasis in Fig. 3.

high UHMWPE wear generated by the large CoCr femoral heads. In the first overview of resurfacing concepts [1], Charnley's small-ball paradigm with polytetrafluoroethylene cups was addressed, but the available wear data on UHMWPE was thought to be equivocal. The largely theoretic concern of higher frictional torques with resurfacing also did not appear to be a clinical issue [8], although this had been a major issue in pioneering MOM designs of the 1960s [9]. Three other concerns included (1) rigid CoCr shells producing stress shielding, (2) fixation with a flexible cement layer being compromised by rigid CoCr shells, and (3) postoperative disruption of blood supply to the head resulting in subsequent osteonecrosis (see the articles by Grigoris et al and Lillikakis et al elsewhere in this issue). Occasional necrosis of the femoral head due to extensive cement penetration has been reported [10], and revision for neck impingement has been an occasional issue [11]. Narrowing of the femoral neck, although of no reported clinical significance, has also appeared as a recognized phenomenon (see the article by Villar elsewhere in this issue).

Although the hemispheric, porous-coated acetabular cup has become standard (see the articles by

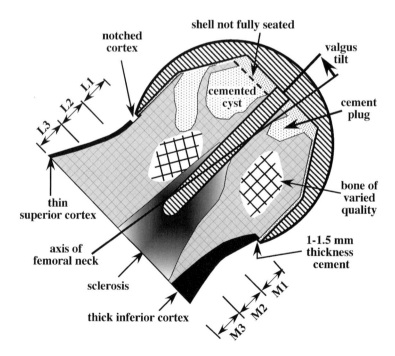

Fig. 3. Schematic of contemporary resurfacing design with a 54-mm diameter femoral shell, a thin cement layer, and a central stem supported by considerably increased bone density (see Fig. 2). Contemporary clinical and finite element analysis studies have defined three regions with increased bone density on superolateral (L1-L3) and inferomedial (M1-M3) neck [17,20].

Grigoris et al and Villar elsewhere in this issue), the long-term survivorship of the femoral shell may not be so clear-cut. The appearance of radiolucent zones and varus migration may still be an issue [12], and the possibilities of neck narrowing or femoral-neck fracture remain of concern [11,13]. The TARA resurfacing shell (Depuy-J&J Inc, Warsaw, IN) was unique in that its long curved stem (Fig. 2) was designed to minimize load bearing in a successful resurfacing and to act as intramedullary fixation if there was a threat of shell migration [14]. Somewhat similar central stems have become universal, either used as "guides" or designed to supplement femoral support by fixation with cement [12], porous ingrowth, or hydroxyapatite coating (see the article by Grigoris et al elsewhere in this issue). Thus, overall, the remaining uncertainties still appear to lie with the femoral side of resurfacing (see Table 2).

Stress remodeling of the proximal femur

Clearly, reaming of the femoral head with installation of a rigid CoCr shell on a flexible matrix of cancellous bone (Fig. 3) results in major changes in how hip loads are transmitted down the femoral neck. Various mathematic models (eg, finite element analysis) have been used to determine whether such stress shielding or stress concentrations could become mechanical causes for failure; that is, producing abnormally low or high stresses and strains [15–17]. Some studies provided comprehensive analyses of variations in hip loading, cup stiffness, bone quality, and bone resorption [18]. It was shown that the normal stress flow from the contact area down through the femoral neck was disrupted (stress shielding) by the MOM resurfacing, and stress concentrations were noted under the rigid CoCr rim. Thus, there have been suggestions that femoral resurfacing could fail due to high, unnatural interface stresses [15,16]. Over the last 30 years of joint-replacement procedures, however, there has been little or no evidence that stress shielding per se has produced adverse clinical effects compared with the ravages of the osteolytic phenomena.

One of the limitations of such mathematic models was their inability to model the complex biologic aspects of failure mechanisms (Table 3). It must also be assumed that any bone remodeling phenomena related to resurfacing during the 1980 to 1990 era were blanketed by the extensive osteolytic changes produced by wear of UHMWPE cups (see Table 1). The clinical history of such cases with UHMWPE cups can be amazingly complex. Even in the same patient, some resurfacings may show complete loss of proximal bone and some may show major bone bridging to the central stem (see Figs. 2 and 3). Thus,

Table 3
Summary of geometric and material assumptions common to computer models of the resurfaced hip

Resurfacing in vivo	FEA assumptions	FEA limitation
Bone behaviour	Linear elastic properties	No
Cement anchored to metal shell	Implant interfaces bonded 100%	No
Bone properties vary directionally	Bone assumed to be isotropic	No
Varied cortical thicknesses	Cortices symmetric	Yes
Thin cement layers (1–1.5 mm)	Varied	No
Varied cement plugs	Not modeled	Yes
Small- versus large-diameter fixation effects	Not modeled	Yes
Interfacial membrane present	Cement bonded	Yes
Varied arthritic bone	Homogeneous	Major
Cystic defects of head	2D-models	Major
Notching of cortex	Not modeled	Major
Varied bone coverage by shell	Not modeled	Major
Varus or valgus shell position	Not modeled	No
Effect of stem size and shape	Varied	No
Stem fixation (none, cement, ingrowth)	Not modeled	Major
Cancellous bone remodeling	Not modeled	Major
Cortical bone remodeling	Not modeled	Major
Shell migration	Not modeled	Yes
Cortical neck narrowing over time	Not modeled	Yes

Abbreviations: 2D, two-dimensional; FEA, finite element analysis.
Data from Refs. [15–17].

it has been very difficult for finite element analysis studies to offer the necessary insight regarding the biologic consequences of bony defects or remodeling to the altered stress state created by the resurfacing intervention (see Table 3).

In vivo, the least complicated clinical case for "stress remodeling" should be evident in patients with avascular necrosis; that is, in young patients with excellent joint anatomy and good-quality bone but with just an isolated segment of collapse in the femoral head. A 10-year review of avascular necrosis cases, however, revealed no evidence of adverse bone remodeling or implant loosening [19]. There was also no evidence of stress shielding, neck narrowing, or progression of osteonecrosis. In addition, the incidence of cup loosening and neck fractures in other MOM resurfacing series has been small, likely indicating that "unnatural stress" effects have had minimal effect (see the article by Grigoris et al elsewhere in this issue). Longitudinal studies of bone remodeling around resurfaced hips from 3 weeks to 2 years showed increasing density of the superior neck over time [20]. At 24 months, the density of the femoral zones was approximately 110% to 140% greater than at 3 weeks. A uniform narrowing of the femoral neck has also been documented [11,21] and may have several origins—perhaps a combination of surgical, mechanical, and biologic insults. In the hemiarthroplasty resurfacing followed-up to 10 years, narrowing of the femoral neck was not observed [19]. Therefore, it is curious that in total MOM resurfacing, neck narrowing has appeared as a fairly common observation (17% incidence by 6 months; see the article by Villar elsewhere in this issue). The causes and consequences of this phenomenon have yet to be elucidated.

Fixation of the metal-on-metal resurfacing

Cement fixation has been used for the metal McKee-Farrar cups (Howmedica-Osteonics Inc, Mahwah, NJ) since 1961. In this regard, it should be noted that such fixation did not prove adequate for the modular CoCr acetabular cups used in the United States [22] or for the alumina ceramic cups [23] and CoCr resurfacing cups used in France (see Table 1). A cemented resurfacing cup was also introduced by McMinn in England and then abandoned (see Table 1). Bone cement, a particularly flexible material (polymethylmethacrylate), has worked well in combination with other flexible materials such as cancellous bone and UHMWPE; however, cement has consistently been found inadequate when anchored to the convex side of rigid acetabular cups. With such hindsight, it is a little surprising that the McKee-Farrar THR, with its cemented rigid cup, could claim reasonable clinical success over 20 years or more [24,25]. From McKee's [4] own series, it is known that more than 40% of the cemented MOM cups migrated 5 mm or more [25]. In contrast, a review of 161 non-cemented Metasul cases followed in 1995–2003 showed no loose cups and no osteolysis [57]. The authors noted their results were greatly superior to the McKee-Farrar system. Thus in complete contrast to the cemented CoCr cup, the porous-coated cup has proved to be a successful implant with its choices of beaded or plasma coatings and adjunct fixation by means of fins, screws, or hydroxyapatite coating (see the articles by Grigoris et al and Lillikakis et al elsewhere in this issue).

Survivorship of the cemented femoral shell appears to be of more concern than the noncemented acetabular cup. One study noted that within 6 years, there were three revisions for fractured necks and seven for loosening of the femoral component (3%). The appearance of femoral stem radiolucencies (4%) was also of concern [12]. The two rigid implant examples that have worked well with cement have been the CoCr femoral condyles of the knee joint and the CoCr femoral shells used in resurfacing (see Table 1). Therefore, it would appear that a thin, flexible layer of cement performs adequately only when keyed to concave surfaces. Thus, most contemporary resurfacing designs have cemented femoral shells, although hydroxyapatite coatings may also be an option (see the article by Villar elsewhere in this issue). As with the earlier resurfacing designs [8], the highest failure rates occurred with the smaller-diameter femoral shells [12]. The greater extent of the fixation interface in larger femoral shells may have protected some patients for greater durations [26]. Thus, if the fixation interface is marginal, then the use of central stems may improve their durability (see Figs. 2 and 3). The question is: What is the bone remodeling response to the combined effect of stem and fixation method? Should the stem be simply a press-fit guide (see Fig. 2) or cemented, porous coated, or even hydroxyapatite coated to enhance its fixation?

In vitro wear studies (metal-on-metal total hip replacement and resurfacing)

Because MOM implants are rigid, the bearings are dimensionally stable, unlike the situation with flexible UHMWPE cups. Thus, the size of the MOM

Table 4
Summary of manufacturing parameters believed to influence the run-in wear and corrosion rates of metal-on-metal bearings

MOM resurfacing parameters	Parameters	Controversial
Diameter effect	38–60 mm	Somewhat
Radial mismatch of ball to cup	25–150 μm	Yes
MOM carbon content	Low, high, hybrid	Somewhat
Alloy type	Cast, wrought	Somewhat
Alloy heat treatments	Solution anneal, hipping	Somewhat
Variability in processing unique to thin shells	Possible	Yes
Sphericity of bearings	<10 μm	No
Surface finish	<30 nm	No
Dimensional accuracy of acetabular cup after insertion	Variable	Possible

contact zone is dictated by manufacturer's specifications (Table 4). Naturally, the diameter of the femoral shell has to be somewhat smaller than that of the acetabular cup; that is, an intentional "mismatch" ("radial" or "diametral clearance"). The mismatch cannot be too small or the bearing may seize due to its geometric irregularities. In the 1960 to 1970 era, the implants were hand finished, and surface irregularities were common [9]. Thus, a small mismatch resulted in stress concentrations around the cup rim, with lubricant starvation and higher frictional torques likely (see the article by Rieker et al elsewhere in this issue) [27]. Laboratory studies of MOM bearings with low radial mismatch also showed that these

would progress with high wear magnitudes [28]. Conversely, the radial mismatch cannot be too large or the contact stresses may become too high and produce exceptionally high wear (see the article by Rieker et al elsewhere in this issue) [2,5,29]. Finite element analysis modeling predicted that decreasing the radial mismatch from 50 to 25 μm had the effect of reducing contact stresses by 50% in 28-mm bearings [30]. The typical radial mismatch in pioneering McKee-Farrar implants was 40 to 150 μm (average, 90 μm) [31]. One simulator study increased the radial mismatch 14-fold, which increased wear rates threefold [32]. Recent studies, however, have predicted that doubling the radial mismatch would

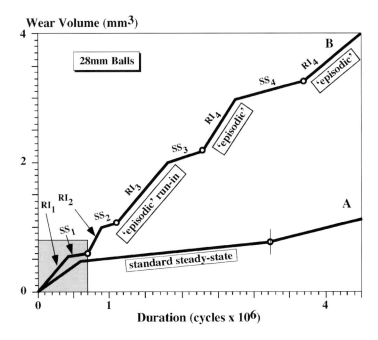

Fig. 4. Two examples of MOM wear responses with 28-mm THRs (Metasul). One THR pair (A) showed classical run-in and steady-state wear pahses [33]. Another apparently identical pair (B) showed an episodic progression of run-in and steady-state phases that overall produced much higher wear magnitude (beginning of renewed 'run-in' phases marked by a circle).

raise wear rates by twofold to fourfold (see the article by Rieker et al elsewhere in this issue). Comparing McKee-Farrar retrievals with Muller THR designs (Sulzer Inc, Berne, Suisse) of similar metallurgy, it was noted that the Muller with the highest radial mismatch (105 μm ± 25 μm) had the lowest wear [28]. Thus the effects of radial mismatch are not well understood and subject to much interpretation.

MOM wear trends are complex because there are generally two discretely different wear rates: "run-in" and "steady-state" phases (Fig. 4) [33]. Run-in wear is high as the two MOM surfaces coadapt; the fluid may turn gray due to the rapidly accumulating metal particulates [34,35]. The run-in phase with 28-mm diameter MOM is accomplished generally within the first 1 million cycles (see Fig. 4; run-in indicated by gray square). It is intuitively obvious that this bedding-in process becomes greater as the initial radial mismatch increases (see the article by Rieker et al elsewhere in this issue). It is also obvious that higher roughness and more out-of-round bearings produce greater volumes of debris during their run-in wear process [36]. Typical out-of-round for ball bearings may be <0.15 μm [37], whereas MOM im-

Table 5
Summary of 28-mm and 36- to 56-mm metal-on-metal wear studies in vitro (ranked by magnitude of run-in wear)

Study	Head diameter (mm)	Mean radial clearance (μm)	Initial Ra (μm)	Carbon content	Volumetric wear rate (mm^3/Mc)		RI/SS ratio
					RI	SS	
Williams et al, 2004 [39]	28	NA	NA	NA	0.13	0.05	2.6
Liao et al, 2004 [40]	28	50	10	High	0.30	0.05	6.0
Firkins et al, 2001 [41]	28	NA	NA	NA	0.31	0.04	7.8
Chan et al, 1999 [42]	28	31	7	High	0.40	0.10	4.0
Chan et al, 1999 [42]	28	~40	14	High	0.60	0.07	8.6
Liao et al, 2004 [40]	28	70	10	High and Low	0.80	0.12	6.7
Roter et al, 2002 [43]	28	NA	NA	High	0.80	0.20	4.0
Scholes et al, 2001 [44]	28	22	8–30	Low	0.90	0.10	9.0
Scholes et al, 2001 [44]	28	40	8–30	Low	0.90	0.75	1.2
Goldsmith et al, 2000 [45]	28	56	8–25	High	1.00	0.45	2.2
Chan et al, 1999 [42]	28	~40	14	Low	1.50	0.13	11.5
Smith et al, 2001 [46]	28	31	5–30	High	1.60	0.54	3.0
Anissian et al, 2001 [33]	28	50	NA	High	2.20	1.00	2.2
Clarke et al, 2000 [47]	28	55	NA	High	2.68	0.97	2.8
Firkins et al, 2001 [41]	28	30	10–20	High	3.09	1.23	2.5
Fisher et al, 2000 [48]	28	NA	NA	NA	3.10	1.60	1.9
Rieker et al, 2001 [49]	28	50	23	High	3.50	1.00	3.5
Bowsher et al, 2004 [50]	28	42	~10	High	4.20	0.92	4.6
Mean wear rate ($mm^3/10^6$ cycles)					1.56	0.52	4.67
Standard deviation					1.3	0.5	2.9
Standard error					0.3	0.1	0.7
95% confidence interval					0.6	0.2	1.4
Liao et al, 2004 [40]	36	70	10	High	0.25	0.08	3.1
Goldsmith et al, 2000 [45]	36	71	6–35	High	1.20	0.36	3.3
Collins et al, 2004 [51]	54	NA	NA·	High	1.91	0.43	4.4
Bowsher et al, 2003 [52]	40	119	15	High	2.20	0.4	5.4
Chan et al, 1996 [36]	45	10–300	25–51	High	5.00	0.6	8.3
Bowsher et al, 2004 [50]	56	142	15	High	7.10	0.32	22.2
Mean wear rate ($mm^3/10^6$ cycles)					2.94	0.37	7.8
Standard deviation					2.6	0.2	7.3
Standard error					1.1	0.1	3
95% confidence interval					2.6	0.2	7.4

Abbreviations: NA, not available; Ra, arithmetic mean assessment of surface roughness; RI, running-in; SS, steady-state.

plants may have a 3- to 10-μm range [36,38]. Many different test conditions were also represented in the various simulator wear studies of the 28-mm MOM bearing (Table 5) [33,36,39–52]. Implant variables included carbon content, alloy processing, radial mismatch, surface roughness, ball sphericity, and alloy heat treatments. Thus, such wear data may not be sufficiently robust to draw definitive conclusions (Fig. 5) [33]. In the authors' 28-mm MOM studies, considerable variability in wear trends for apparently identical 28-mm THRs was noted. Sometimes the classic run-in and steady-state wear patterns were evident (see Fig. 4; trend A). The authors also observed a contrary wear behavior that they termed an *episodic run-in* wear trend (see Fig. 4; trend B). Possibly these repeated, run-in wear events occurred due to the MOM ball–cup relationship not being established precisely each time in the wear machine. Such episodic run-in wear may have implications for in vitro and in vivo variability with MOM. Thus, in overview, it may be adequate to simply point out that the 28-mm MOM wear rates have been low, with run-in and steady-state wear averaging <4 mm^3/Mc and <1.6 mm^3/Mc, respectively (see Table 5). This wear is still at least one order of magnitude less than that observed during the comparable era with UHMWPE cups.

Wear rates have been relatively low using the larger diameters typical of resurfacing, with averages of <7.1 mm^3/Mc and <0.6 mm^3/Mc for run-in and steady-state, respectively (see Table 5). Therefore, as a first approximation, resurfacing run-in wear-rates averaged twice those of 28-mm THRs. Comparing diameter effects, there appears to be a linear trend for run-in wear to increase with ball diameter (see Fig. 5; 36- to 56-mm range), which represents a fourfold wear increase overall. The corresponding steady-state wear appeared to be about the same or marginally less than with the 28-mm MOM. There have been many theoretic studies predicting that the larger-diameter MOM will have improved "fluid-film" lubrication and therefore benefit from reduced wear rates [47]. Such theoretic predictions appear contradictory to the evidence presented here for run-in wear; there is certainly room for dispute, even under steady-state laboratory conditions.

It has been noted that worn surfaces on retrieved UHMWPE and crosslinked polyethylene cups appeared smooth to the eye [53,54], as did the high-wearing Hylamer cups (Depuy-J&J, Warsaw, IN) [55]. Similarly, the worn surfaces of MOM appeared "polished" to the eye; however, from a microscopic point of view, retrieved McKee-Farrar THRs demonstrated a central (polar) region and, in some cases, a peripheral worn area (Fig. 6). A retrieval study of 22 McKee THRs noted that those with more peripheral wear had an average lifespan of only 9 years compared with those with polar wear that averaged

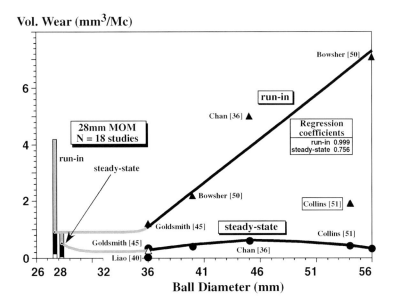

Fig. 5. Comparison of run-in and steady-state wear trends (Table 5). Note that direct comparison of large versus 28-mm ball diameter wear-rates is made difficult by confounding variations in implant and test parameters, notably radial mismatch and serum concentrations. (*Data from* Refs. [33,36,39–52].)

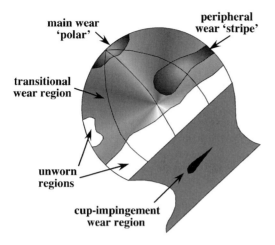

main wear
'polar'

peripheral
wear 'stripe'

transitional
wear region

unworn
regions

cup-impingement
wear region

Fig. 6. Schematic of wear patterns on a McKee-Farrar femoral head retrieved at 4 years including main-wear 'polar' region on dome, peripheral-wear 'stripe' near the equator (Modes-1, -2), and impingement wear on femoral neck (Mode-4). The depth of stripe wear was estimated to be 1 μm. (*Adapted from* Walker PS, Salvati E, Hotzler RK. The wear on removed McKee-Farrar total hip prostheses. J Bone Joint Surg [Am] 1974;56:95.)

13 years [56]. In cases with MOM impingement, a more severe stripe wear has been noted [68,69]. Recent simulator studies using microseparation test modes have also produced stripe wear in MOM bearings [58]. Such MOM stripe wear appeared identical in shape, size, and location to those described in the authors' studies of ceramic THRs retrieved after 15 to 22 years' use [59–62]. This finding should not come as a surprise because such "edge" effects of rigid acetabular cups have been documented for over 3 decades. It is worth reiterating that a series of 345 non-cemented Metasul hips begun in 1995 continues to show excellent clinical results [57].

Run-in and steady-state wear in patients (surrogate studies of ion levels)

Looking at the worst-case scenario in patients, the overall risk of MOM bearings can be characterized by the potential modes of debris production [63]. Mode-1 wear is normal wear between the CoCr ball and cup (Fig. 7a). It is also intuitive that unlike the flexible UHMWPE cup, the CoCr cup has the potential to create stripe wear on the opposing ball surface due to the stress-enhancement effect of its rigid

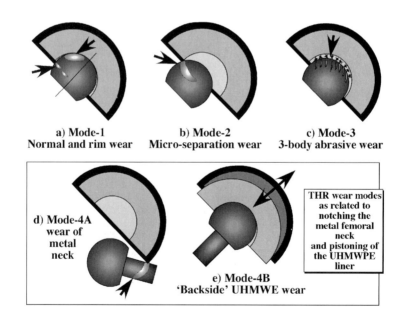

a) Mode-1
Normal and rim wear

b) Mode-2
Micro-separation wear

c) Mode-3
3-body abrasive wear

d) Mode-4A
wear of
metal
neck

e) Mode-4B
'Backside' UHMWE wear

THR wear modes
as related to
notching the
metal femoral
neck
and pistoning of
the UHMWPE
liner

Fig. 7. Possible wear modes in hip arthroplasty. (*a*) Mode-1 wear: normal polar region and some equatorial peripheral regions. (*b*) Mode-2 wear: cup rim effect, producing stripe wear at or above equator on femoral ball. (*c*) Mode-3 wear: third-body abrasion of ball and cup. (*d*) Mode-4a wear: rim notching of the femoral neck with cup abrasion. (*e*) Mode-4b wear: 'backside wear' due to micromotion of liner. (*Adapted from* McKellop HA, Campbell P, Park SH, et al. The origin of submicron polyethylene wear debris in total hip arthroplasty. Clin Orthop 1995;311:3–20.)

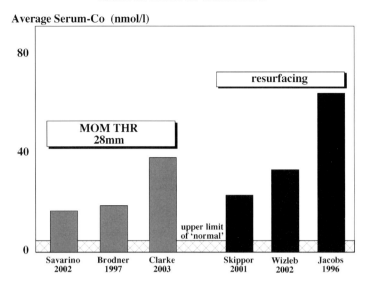

Fig. 8. Comparisons of serum-cobalt (serum-Co) levels in MOM patients. The estimate of maximum "normal" concentrations for serum cobalt and serum chromium is shown by the hatched area. (*Data from* Clarke MT, Lee PTH, Arora A, Villar N. Levels of metal ions after small- and large-diameter metal-on-metal hip arthroplasty. J Bone Joint Surg [Br] 2003;85:913–7.)

rim (see Figs. 6 and 7a). The effect of a rigid CoCr cup rim would be much more severe on femoral balls made of soft materials, and this is the main reason that polymeric femoral balls have never met with success inside rigid metal cups [64–66]. Mode-2 wear anticipates that microseparation during the swing phase of gait [67] or other subluxation episodes will create additional impact of cup rim at heelstrike and thereby promote a severe form of stripe wear (see Fig. 7b) [58]. Mode-3 wear occurs with

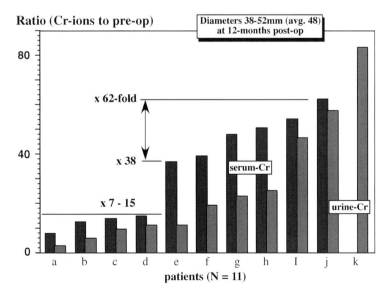

Fig. 9. Serum and urine concentrations of metal ions at 12 months ranked in increasing order for resurfacing patients. avg, average; Cr, chromium; post-op, postoperative; pre-op, preoperative. (*Data from* Skipor AK, Campbell PA, Patterson LM, et al. Serum and urine metal levels in patients with metal-on-metal surface arthroplasty. J Mater Sci Mater Med 2002;13(12): 1227–34.)

third-body, abrasive contaminants (see Fig. 7c). One of the consequences of THR designs is that their metallic cups can produce metal-to-metal impingement (Mode-4A); the resulting cup/neck-notching and metallosis have had dramatic consequences [55,68]. This femoral neck to cup impingement may present clinically as the "squeaking hip" syndrome in a patient [43,69]. Impingement can also happen with resurfacing but will likely be against the bone of the femoral neck. Mode-4B wear involves the "backside" wear that may be unique to suboptimal fixation of the liner in modular THR cups (see Fig. 7e).

Normal MOM wear rates are too minute to be identified radiographically. Microscopically, the MOM wear debris is much less conspicuous in the joint tissues than UHMWPE debris and usually found in mononuclear phagocytes close to the vicinity of blood vessels transitioning between the inner synovial lining and the outer joint capsule [70]. Histology of retrieved tissues shows extensive necrosis within the newly formed synovial membrane, with a diffuse lymphoplasmacytic infiltrate especially evident around the small blood vessels. This tissue response is considered a typical reaction to MOM wear products and denotes a local immune response to cobalt and chromium [71–73]. The metal particles have been easily identified in periarticular tissues that were colored black or gray but not in more normal-appearing tissues [74]. It has been estimated that CoCr particles numbering up to 2×10^{14} were released per year with 28-mm THRs [74]. This estimate represents approximately 200 million particles released for each step that the patient takes on a MOM bearing. Because the CoCr particulate generally has a median size smaller than 50 nm, the resulting surface area of metal exposed to body fluids is large [72]. As a result of such MOM wear characteristics, surrogate wear comparisons have been made by monitoring the cobalt and chromium ion levels from the patient's red blood cells, serum, and urine [75]; only recently have testing protocols become stringent enough to allow discrimination at parts per billion [76]. The periarticular release of such large quantities of minute particles raises the question of how fast will the corrosion of such trapped particles be translated into elevated ion concentrations that can be measurable in the patient's serum or urine?

Because THR designs (28 mm) have the most risk of impingement and dislocation (see Figs. 1 and 7) and are reputed to produce more volumetric wear [77], the authors hypothesized that the THR cases would show the highest ion concentrations. As an overview of the published median values, the

authors' first observation was that the THR patients displayed less ion concentrations than resurfacing patients regardless of implants used and follow-up durations (Fig. 8). Comparison of MOM resurfacing cases (Conserve Plus, Wright Medical Technology Inc, Tennessee; see the article by Grigoris et al elsewhere in this issue) showed varied patterns of ion release in serum and urine over the first 12 months (Fig. 9) [78]. One patient profile showed that ion levels could be elevated 90-fold at 6 months and then drop to a 40-fold elevation by the 12-month review. This finding suggested that a steady-state wear phase had been achieved within 6 months. A contrasting patient profile attained a 20-fold elevation at 6 months but increased further to a 40-fold elevation at 12 months, suggesting that MOM wear was still increasing. Overall comparisons of serum chromium and urine chromium levels at 12 months showed two groups of resurfacing results, one with serum chromium elevated from 7 to 15 fold and the other elevated from 38 to 62 fold (Fig. 9). There was no

Concentration (nmol/l)

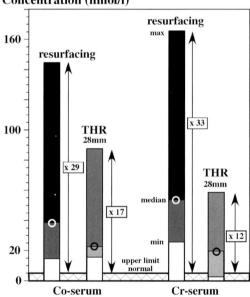

Fig. 10. MOM ion levels in patients matched with resurfacing and THR (56-month clinical course; median, 16 months). The minimum ion concentrations are indicated by white bars, median values are indicated by circles, and maximum ranges are shown in black. The estimate of maximum "normal" concentrations for serum cobalt (Co-serum) and serum chromium (Cr-serum) is shown by the hatched area. (*Data from* Clarke MT, Lee PTH, Arora A, Villar N. Levels of metal ions after small- and large-diameter metal-on-metal hip arthroplasty. J Bone Joint Surg [Br] 2003; 85:913–7.)

apparent differentiation by age, sex, or ball diameter, perhaps due to the small number of patients with complete data (N = 11). Because these cases were all resurfacing cases, the differences could not have been due to Mode-4 types of wear. Therefore, the authors' postulate that the patients with low ion levels had achieved steady-state wear and those with higher ion levels were still in their run-in phase. The reason for the latter could be that patients had an inferior radial mismatch (see the article by Rieker et al elsewhere in this issue) or they possibly experienced episodic run-in wear (see Fig. 4) for some other reason.

A THR study (28 mm) showed peak ion concentrations at 50-fold and 100-fold over controls during a 4-year study [71]. With one of the THR designs (SIKOMET), the concentrations dropped markedly beyond 15 months, apparently signaling that the run-in wear was over. Surprisingly, the ion levels began to rise again by the fourth year of study. In contrast, with a second THR design (Metasul, Zimmer-CenterPulse, Austin, TX), the ion concentrations were high for 3 years and dropped only toward the fourth postoperative year. The study concluded that even at 4 years, the alloy concentrations were markedly elevated above postoperative levels. Labo-

ratory studies of large clearances in MOM have indeed shown such a protracted run-in wear phase (see the article by Rieker et al elsewhere in this issue). Comparison of patients carefully matched with MOM resurfacing and THR implants also showed that the ion concentrations were higher with larger ball size (Fig. 10).

One way of assessing temporal wear/corrosion effects is to measure ion concentrations in patients before and just after exercise. Five patients with 28-mm Metasul THRs were matched to five patients with the Cormet-2000 design and five patients with the Birmingham Hip Resurfacing (Fig. 11) [79]. The patients were matched by age, sex, body mass index, time after surgery, and the number of steps taken during the organized program. The patients had also been instructed to not exercise extensively in the week prior. The subjects wore pedometers and walked or ran at their own pace for 1 hour in a playing field. Blood samples were taken before, just after, and 1 hour after their exercise. In terms of effect due to increased activity level, 50% of the patients showed peak elevations in cobalt and chromium ions immediately after exercising and the remainder had higher peaks 1 hour later. The ion increase was in the

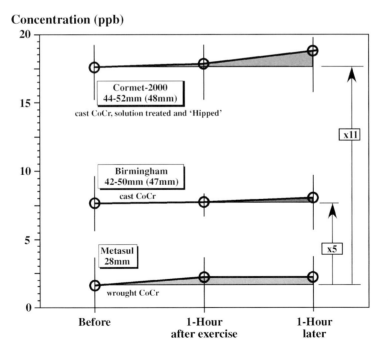

Fig. 11. Ranking of metal ions in blood from patients with three types of MOM implants before and after a 1-hour exercise regime. (*Data from* Takahashi T, Kuiper JH, Gile S, et al. Effect of exercise on metal levels in patients with three different metal-on-metal hip replacements. In: Proceedings of the American Academy of Orthopaedic Surgeons. San Francisco, California. American Academy of Orthopaedic Surgeons; 2004. p. 71.)

5% to 40% range for Metasul patients and 5% to 16% for resurfacing. Compared with healthy volunteers as controls, the ion levels with the 28-mm Metasul THR were elevated threefold to fivefold on average. With resurfacing, the ion levels were elevated 8 to 17 fold higher for cobalt and 17 to 32 fold higher for chromium. This study clearly reflected major effects of variables of materials, design, diameters, and tolerances using three different MOM bearings in a carefully matched patient population. The biggest difference in ion concentrations was due to implant type, with the Birmingham Hip Resurfacing and Cormet-2000 bearings showing fivefold and 11-fold higher levels, respectively (see Fig. 11). Thus, there were some interesting consistencies in these clinical data regarding MOM ball size effects and some amazing design and follow-up effects that remain to be explored more fully in subsequent MOM studies.

Summary

The current era of MOM resurfacing has benefited from the 40-year history of THRs (see Table 1). The unique value of the thin, acetabular cup technology used in contemporary THR bearings has been particularly timely for resurfacing (Table 6) (see article by Lilikakis et al elsewhere in this issue) [12,38,57,78,80–83]; however, even with a 34-year history, the efficacy of the cemented femoral shell has clearly been overshadowed by UHMWPE-driven osteolysis of prior designs. Nevertheless, cement fixation of the femoral shell appears satisfactory, as indicated by the success of current MOM resurfacing series (Table 7), although fixation may be marginal in some patients fitted with smaller diameters of femoral shell [26]. For increased fixation opportunity, the central stem first used some 40 years ago, even before the TARA concept, has now become standard for adjunct femoral alignment and fixation. Thus, the remaining challenges include the long-term success of the femoral resurfacing and potential risk of adverse MOM wear conditions.

The narrowing of the femoral neck, although not a clinical problem, remains a perplexing biologic phenomenon. In canine resurfacing models, a cortical thickening accompanied by an overall thinning of the femoral neck within 8 months of follow-up was noted [84,85]. Similar cortical thickening and neck narrowing has been reported in various resurfacing series. A "biomechanical" explanation may be that the bone responds to the altered stress conditions by adding sclerotic bone distal to the implant and that this "reinforcement" in the femoral neck results in decreasing dimensions (see Fig. 2; see radiograph of left hip). This situation, however, should be identical in hemiresurfacing patients who share many of the features of MOM resurfacing (Table 8) [33,36,39–52]. The presence of a central stem protruding distally may significantly alter the stress state as bone remodeling continues around it (see Figs. 2 and 3). Although femoral resurfacing appears to be a deceptively simple geometric problem, the complexity of such bone remodeling phenomena has remained outside the scope of any computer model (see Table 3).

Table 6
Summary of contemporary metal-on-metal resurfacing results (ranked by age of patients)

MOM study	Implant	No. of hips	Age			Duration			REV	REV%
			MIN	MAX	AVG	MIN	MAX	AVG		
Beaule 2004 [80]	Resurfacing	94	15	40	34	3	6.8	4	3	3.2
Kim 2004 [81]	THR (28)	70	17	49	37	5	9	7	1	1.4
Daniel 2004 [13]	Resurfacing	384	27	55	48	1	8.2	3.3	1	0.3
Grigoris et al 2005, this issue	Resurfacing	200	22	72	48	NA	3	NA	0	0.0
Amstutz et al 2004 [10]	Resurfacing	400	15	77	48	2	6	3.5	13	3.3
Skipor et al 2002 [78]	Resurfacing	25	28	62	49	0.25	1	NA		Ion study
Lilikakis et al 2005, this issue	Resurfacing	70	23	73	51	2	3	2	1	1.4
Clarke et al 2003 [38]	Resurfacing (THR28)	22 (22)	39	77	53	0.5	4.5	1.7	NA	Ion study
Brodner 2005 [82]	THR (28)	60	13	85	57	3	6	4.4	NA	Ion study
Long et al [57]	THR (28)	127	20	84	72	5	11	6	4	3.2
Glyn-Jones 2004 [83]	Resurfacing	22	NA	60	NA	0.25	3	NA	NA	RSA study

Abbreviations: AVG, average; MAX, maximum; MIN, minimum; NA, not available; REV, revision cases; RSA, radiostereometry analysis of implant migration.

Table 7
Possible scenarios to explain the uniform thinning of the femoral neck following resurfacing arthroplasty, including mechanical and biological effects

Parameter	Hemiarthroplasty	MOM resurfacing
Surgical impact to head	NA	NA
Femoral-shell design	NA	NA
Femoral fixation	NA	NA
Abnormal cortical stresses	NA	NA
Abnormal cancellous-bone stresses	NA	NA
Surgical impact to acetabulum	None	Longer operation
More vascular compromise	Normal	Yes
Mode-2 impingement	None	Yes
Wear particulates	Minimal	Yes
MOM ions	Minimal	Yes
Patient activity	Resumed	Resumed

Abbreviation: NA, not available.

Thus, the risk-to-benefit ratios of the latest designs of femoral shells must come from careful clinical study (Box 1).

Wear studies of MOM bearings were greatly accelerated with the introduction of the 28-mm Metasul THR in 1988. Although many variations in alloys and simulator test conditions were used to

Table 8
Suggested knowledge base for deciphering metal-on-metal wear responses in vitro and in vivo

MOM knowledge base ("pristine" simulator conditions)	Reference
Larger MOM diameters have higher run-in wear	[37,45,52,56][a]
Larger radial mismatches have higher run-in wear	Rieker et al, this issue
Rougher MOM surfaces have higher run-in wear	[36]
MOM roughness (<30 nm) is reduced by wear (Ra<10 nm)	Rieker et al, this issue
Larger out-of-round MOM will have higher run-in wear	[80]
Run-in wear may endure <1 million cycles to >4 million cycles	Rieker et al, this issue
Steady-state wear may be reduced threefold to fivefold on average	[33,36,39–52][b]
Larger MOM bearings expected to reduce steady-state wear	[33,36,39–52][a]

Abbreviation: Ra, assessment of surface roughness by arithmetic average.
 [a] See Fig. 5.
 [b] See Table 5.

Box 1. Technologic benefits accruing to metal-on-metal resurfacing in 2005

MOM manufacturing technology much superior to prior 4 decades
Porous-coated acetabular cup provides extremely successful fixation mode
CoCr acetabular cup provides space-saving MOM bearing
Femoral stem provides adjunct alignment and fixation benefits
CoCr shell cement fixation successful at 3–6 years' average follow-up
MOM wear rate significantly less than UHMWPE
MOM cup-neck impingement (THR) obviated with resurfacing (Mode-4A)
Backside wear obviated with nonmodular resurfacing cups (Mode-4B)

study such 28-mm bearings (see Table 5), it was encouraging to find that the maximum wear was <4 mm^3/Mc. This wear was at least one order of magnitude less than with the UHMWPE cups used in the 1980 to 1990 era. The importance played by manufacturing parameters such as surface roughness, sphericity, and radial mismatch during the run-in wear of MOM bearings has been shown (see the article by Rieker et al elsewhere in this issue). Such wide variations in 28-mm MOM wear-rates (see Fig. 5) may also indicate that the data for or against variations in CoCr metallurgy are not yet convincing. Published clinical studies have tended to favor the high-carbide alloys [13,71,86]. Thus, it may be advisable to subject MOM bearings to more-severe testing regimes evaluating run-in and steady-state conditions to provide better discrimination of such proposed benefits.

Of concern to the surgeon is the fate of the trillions of metal particulates dispersed into the joint space each year [74], with some portion transported to the lymph nodes, liver, and spleen and some portion readily excreted [87,88]. There has also been an indication that the highest tissue levels of metal ions are not found periarticular but are found in lymph nodes and bone marrow [89]. There have also been many clinical reports of elevated metal concentrations in blood, serum, and urine [90], thus raising the issues of periprosthetic, lymphocytic vasculitis, fibrinoid necrosis, and fibrous intimal proliferation that can occur with MOM, even in the absence of overt metallosis [71,76,86]. It has been suggested that patients with a history of third-body wear, impingement, and dislocation problems with MOM bearings have higher wear and more-elevated ion concentrations [70,91]. It has also been pointed out that such ion concentrations are of a low magnitude (of the order of parts per billion) and, to date, have been of little clinical consequence (see Figs. 8–11) [92]. The authors' particular interest at Loma Linda University Medical Center is that routine patient monitoring of cobalt and chromium ion levels provides a surrogate method of wear detection that will be of great assistance to tribologic studies of many controversial wear-related parameters (see Table 4).

The current topical question is What is the role for the large-diameter MOM bearings given such concerns over the body burden of metal particulates and metal ion concentrations? The apparent disconnect in wear performance between the 28-mm diameter MOM and the larger diameters is perplexing (see Fig. 6). Clearly, the confounding factors have not been adequately addressed in such wear studies (see Table 4). Classical teaching is that the larger the ball, the superior its fluid-film lubrication. Therefore, wear rates and levels of metal ions released were predicted to be lower with larger-diameter bearings [31,93]. The analyses of MOM wear performance, however, is additionally complicated due to many variations in alloys and design tolerances (see the article by Rieker et al elsewhere in this issue). An additional complexity generally underappreciated in such in vitro studies is that larger ball diameters may perpetuate frictional heating that promotes protein degradation. Such precipitates minimize the actual wear processes between metal surfaces [47,94]. Thus, in overview from the literature, there appears to be a significant wear penalty with the larger-diameter balls as assessed during run-in (see Fig. 6). This finding is contrary to

previous predictions that two orders of magnitude of reduction in wear would be achievable by increasing femoral diameters up to 36 mm [93]. Thus, classic fluid-film theory and experimental results appeared to be on a contradictory course from the authors' perspective. Given the multifactorial nature of such in vitro wear studies (see Table 5) and frequently contradictory conclusions [72], it is necessary to go to the clinical model to review what patients are actually experiencing.

The starting hypothesis for our review was that patients with the small-diameter THR would have higher risk of impingement wear [68,69] and thus reveal the maximum metal concentrations in serum and urine. It was therefore interesting that the resurfacing designs appeared to show the highest metal concentrations (Figs. 8–11). Although these data may be imprecise with considerable overlap, the authors did not find any study that showed that the 28-mm Metasul THR bearings had higher CoCr levels than resurfacing series. Therefore, simulator and clinical studies appear to directly challenge the assumption that larger MOM bearings offer improved lubrication and reduced bioburden of cobalt and chromium ions (Table 9). There may be several reasons for this apparent disconnect between theoretic and wear results with the big-ball MOM paradigm. It is clear that the resurfacing designs have been manufactured with a larger radial mismatch between ball and cup. This feature alone can result in higher MOM run-in wear and for much longer durations in patients—perhaps 3 to 5 years or more (see Table 9 and the article by Rieker et al elsewhere in this issue). This mismatch could be the dominant cause for the observed higher wear with resurfacing because the studies of metal ion concentrations have follow-ups to only 6 years (see Table 6). Thus variations in re-

Table 9
Possible scenarios to explain

Resurfacing parameters	Hypotheses for higher ion concentrations	References
Processing and dimensional tolerances	Not as good as mature 28-mm bearing technology	Daniel 2004 [13] [28,79,96]
Big balls = larger sliding distance and higher wear	Contradicts fluid-film lubrication theories	[6][a]
Deformation of cups during insertion	Out-of-round condition creates greater wear	[36]; Rieker et al, this issue
Porous-coated acetabular shells	Easy ingress for particles = third-body wear	[97]
(1) Large radial mismatch	Run-in wear phase lasts up to 4 years	Rieker et al, this issue
(2) Large radial mismatch	Run-in wear rate perpetuates (no steady-state phase)	[28]
High-demand patient	Overstresses the MOM passive surface layer	[33][b]
Change in patient activities (eg, sports)	New wear direction, new run-in wear phase	[33][b]

[a] Charnley paradigm (see Fig. 1).
[b] Episodic run-in wear (see Fig. 4).

surfacing metallurgy and radical mismatch may be two reasons why individual patients can exhibit ion concentrations 40 to 80 fold higher than are typical for MOM medians (see Fig. 9) [95]. Nevertheless, there may be other compelling arguments that could promote episodic run-in wear with MOM bearings (see Fig. 7), particularly in the younger, more-at-risk patients (see Table 6) [96,97]. In three sets of retrieved MOM resurfacing (diameter 40–52 mm: radial mismatch 115–133 μm), the highest wear was attributed to subluxation episodes causing peripheral wear stripes [11]. However the appearance of 'stripe' wear is a known consequence when using ceramic THR [62,98]. Many MOM studies have concluded that such 'peripheral' or 'stripe' wear was a consequence of sub-optimal or 'negative' clearances [29, 31,99]. In contrast, simulator studies have produced such 'stripe' wear on contemporary MOM designs with an order of magnitude increase in wear [58]. Therefore, the stress-concentration effect of the CoCr cup edge [30] also may be an under recognized consequence for MOM wear. In addition, there were major differences between designs and manufacturers (see Fig. 11), so it may be difficult to determine from current data whether the wear response is solely related to MOM diameter or how other factors may interact to influence wear. With the advent of THR diameters in the 38- to 60-mm range (see Table 1) and with their exceedingly large head-to-neck ratios (see Fig. 1), it will be even more compelling to compare ion concentrations released by small- and large-diameter MOM bearings. It is therefore important that surrogate wear methods continue to evolve from current research into valid clinical tools for monitoring metal ion concentrations circulating in the body.

Acknowledgments

The authors are grateful to K. Lester of Fresno Orthopedics, P. Williams of the Department of Orthopedics at Loma Linda University Medical Center, and P. Beaule and P. Campbell of the Joint Replacement Institute, Orthopedic Hospital, Los Angeles for their editorial assistance.

References

[1] Clarke IC. Symposium on surface replacement arthroplasty of the hip. Bbiomechanics: mutifactorial design choices—an essential compromise? Orthop Clin N Am 1982;13(4):681–707.

[2] Amstutz HC, Grigoris P. Metal on metal bearings in hip arthroplasty. Clin Orthop 1996;32(Suppl):S11–34.

[3] Clarke IC. Wear-screening and joint simulation studies vs materials selection and prosthesis design. Crc Crit Rev Biomed Eng 1982;8(1):29–91.

[4] McKee GK, Chen SC. The statistics of the McKee-Farrar method of total hip replacement. Clin Orthop 1973;95:26–33.

[5] Amstutz HC, Campbell P, McKellop H, et al. Metal on metal total hip replacement workshop consensus document. Clin Orthop 1996;329(Suppl):S297–303.

[6] Charnley J, Kamangar A, Longfield MD. The optimum size of prosthetic heads in relation to the wear of plastic sockets in total replacement of the hip. Med Biol Eng 1969;7(1):31–9.

[7] Clarke IC, Good V, Anissian L, et al. Charnley wear model for validation of hip simulators—ball diameter versus polytetrafluoroethylene and polyethylene wear. Proc Inst Mech Eng [H] 1997;211(1):25–36.

[8] Mai MT, Schmalzried TP, Dorey FJ, et al. The contribution of frictional torque to loosening at the cement-bone interface in Tharies hip replacements. J Bone Joint Surg [Am] 1996;78(4):505–11.

[9] Wilson JN, Scales JT. Loosening of total hip replacements with cement fixation. Clinical findings and laboratory studies. Clin Orthop 1970;72:145–60.

[10] Amstutz HC, Beaule PE, Dorey FJ, et al. Metal-on-metal hybrid surface arthroplasty: two to six-year follow-up study. J Bone Joint Surg [Am] 2004;86(1):28–39.

[11] Beaule PE, Le Duff M, Campbell P, et al. Metal-on-metal surface arthroplasty with a cemented femoral component: a 7–10 year follow-up study. J Arthroplasty 2004;19(8 Suppl 3):17–22.

[12] Amstutz HC, Campbell PA, Le Duff MJ. Fracture of the neck of the femur after surface arthroplasty of the hip. J Bone Joint Surg [Am] 2004;86(9):1874–7.

[13] Daniel J, Pynsent PB, McMinn DJ. Metal-on-metal resurfacing of the hip in patients under the age of 55 years with osteoarthritis. J Bone Joint Surg [Br] 2004;86(2):177–84.

[14] Townley CO. Hemi and total articular replacement arthroplasty of the hip with the fixed femoral cup. Orthop Clin N Am 1982;13(4):869–94.

[15] Shybut GT, Askew MJ, Hori RY, et al. Theoretical and experimental studies of femoral stresses following surface replacement hip arthroplasty. Proc Inst Med Chic 1980;33(3):95–106.

[16] Huiskes R, Strens PH, van Heck J, et al. Interface stresses in the resurfaced hip. Finite element analysis of load transmission in the femoral head. Acta Orthop Scand 1985;56(6):474–8.

[17] Watanabe Y, Shiba N, Matsuo S, et al. Biomechanical study of the resurfacing hip arthroplasty: finite element analysis of the femoral component. J Arthroplasty 2000;15(4):505–11.

[18] Huiskes R, Strens P, Vroemen W, et al. Post-loosening mechanical behavior of femoral resurfacing prostheses. Clin Mater 1990;6(1):37–55.

[19] Grecula MJ, Thomas JA, Kreuzer SW. Impact of implant design on femoral head hemiresurfacing arthroplasty. Clin Orthop 2004;418:41–7.

[20] Kishida Y, Sugano N, Nishii T, et al. Preservation of the bone mineral density of the femur after surface replacement of the hip. J Bone Joint Surg [Br] 2004; 86(2):185–9.

[21] McMinn D, Treacy R, Lin K, et al. Metal on metal surface replacement of the hip. Experience of the McMinn prothesis. Clin Orthop 1996;329(Suppl): S89–98.

[22] Harris WH. Advances in total hip arthroplasty. The metal-backed acetabular component. Clin Orthop 1984;183:4–11.

[23] Sedel L. Evolution of alumina-on-alumina implants: a review. Clin Orthop 2000;379:48–54.

[24] Schmalzried TP, Fowble VA, Ure KJ, et al. Metal on metal surface replacement of the hip. Technique, fixation, and early results. Clin Orthop 1996;329(Suppl): S106–14.

[25] August AC, Aldam CH, Pynsent PB. The McKee-Farrar hip arthroplasty. A long-term study. J Bone Joint Surg [Br] 1986;68(4):520–7.

[26] Beaule PE, Dorey FJ, LeDuff M, et al. Risk factors affecting outcome of metal-on-metal surface arthroplasty of the hip. Clin Orthop 2004;418:87–93.

[27] Rieker CB, Kottig P, Schon R. Clinical wear performance of metal-on-metal hip arthroplasties. In: Jacobs TL, Craig TL, editors. Alternative bearing surfaces in total joint replacement. American Society for Testing and Materials. p. 144–56.

[28] Schmidt M, Weber H, Schon R. Cobalt chromium molybdenum metal combination for modular hip prostheses. Clin Orthop 1996;329(Suppl):S35–47.

[29] McKellop H, Park SH, Chiesa R, et al. In vivo wear of three types of metal on metal hip prostheses during two decades of use. Clin Orthop 1996;329(Suppl): S128–40.

[30] Verdonschot N, Vena P, Stolk J, et al. Effects of metal-inlay thickness in polyethylene cups with metal-on-metal bearings. Clin Orthop 2002;404:353–61.

[31] Yew A, Jagatia M, Ensaff H, et al. Analysis of contact mechanics in McKee-Farrar metal-on-metal hip implants. Proc Inst Mech Eng [H] 2003;217(5):333–40.

[32] Scott RA, Schroeder D. The effect of radial mismatch on the wear of metal on metal hip prosthesis: a hip simulator study. In: Proceedings of the Annual Meeting of the Orthopaedic Research Society. San Francisco, California. Rosemont (IL): Orthopaedic Research Society; 1997. p. 764.

[33] Anissian HL, Stark A, Good V, et al. The wear pattern in metal-on-metal hip prostheses. J Biomed Mater Res 2001;58(6):673–8.

[34] Saikko V, Nevalainen J, Revitzer H, et al. Metal release from total hip articulations in vitro: substantial from CoCr/CoCr, negligible from CoCr/PE and alumina/PE. Acta Orthop Scand 1998;69(5): 449–54.

[35] McKellop H, Amstutz H, Lu B, et al. A hip simulator study of the wear of large diameter, metal-on-metal hip surface replacements. In: Proceedings of the 27th Annual Meeting of the Society of Biomaterials. Saint Paul, Minnesota. Minneapolis (MN): Society for Biomaterials; 2001. p. 339.

[36] Chan FW, Bobyn JD, Medley JB, et al. Engineering issues and wear performance of metal on metal hip implants. Clin Orthop 1996;333:96–107.

[37] Schey JA. Systems view of optimizing metal on metal bearings. Clin Orthop 1996;329(Suppl):S115–27.

[38] Clarke MT, Lee PT, Arora A, et al. Levels of metal ions after small- and large-diameter metal-on-metal hip arthroplasty. J Bone Joint Surg [Br] 2003;85(6): 913–7.

[39] Williams S, Stewart TD, Ingham E, et al. Metal-on-metal bearing wear with different swing phase loads. J Biomed Mater Res 2004;70B(2):233–9.

[40] Liao YS, Hanes M, Fryman C, et al. Effects of head size, clearance and start-stop protocol on wear of metal-on-metal hip bearings. In: Transactions 7th World Biomaterials Congress. 2004. p. 82.

[41] Firkins PJ, Tipper JL, Saadatzadeh MR, et al. Quantitative analysis of wear and wear debris from metal-on-metal hip prostheses tested in a physiological hip joint simulator. Biomed Mater Eng 2001;11(2): 143–57.

[42] Chan FW, Bobyn JD, Medley JB, et al. The Otto Aufranc Award. Wear and lubrication of metal-on-metal hip implants. Clin Orthop 1999;369:10–24.

[43] Roter G, Medley J, Cheng N, et al. Intermittent motion: a clinically significant protocol for metal-metal hip simulator testing. In: Transactions 48th Annual Meeting Orthopaedic Research Society, Dallas, Texas. Rosemont (IL): Orthopaedic Research Society; 2002. p. 100.

[44] Scholes SC, Green SM, Unsworth A. The wear of metal-on-metal total hip prostheses measured in a hip simulator. Proc Inst Mech Eng Vol 215, part H. p. 523–30.

[45] Goldsmith AA, Dowson D, Isaac GH, et al. A comparative joint simulator study of the wear of metal-on-metal and alternative material combinations in hip replacements. Proc Inst Mech Eng [H] 2000; 214(1):39–47.

[46] Smith SL, Dowson D, Goldsmith AA. The effect of femoral head diameter upon lubrication and wear of metal-on-metal total hip replacements. Proc Inst Mech Eng [H] 2001;215(2):161–70.

[47] Clarke I, Good V, Williams P, et al. Hip simulator wear trends in polymeric, all-metal, and all-ceramic bearings with water and serum "lubrication." In: Ura A, editor. The Proceedings of the International Tribology Conference, Nagasaki, Japan. Tokyo: Ohsato Printing Center Co.; 2000. p. 1497–502.

[48] Fisher J, Besong AA, Firkins PJ, et al. Comparative wear and debris generation in UHMWPE on ceramic, metal on metal and ceramic on ceramic hip protheses. In: Transactions 46th Annual Meeting Orthopaedic Research Society, Orlando, Florida.

Rosemont (IL): Orthopaedic Research Society; 2004. p. 587.

[49] Rieker C, Konrad R, Schon R. In vitro comparison of the two hard-hard articulations for total hip replacements. Proc Inst Mech Eng [H] 2001;215(2): 153–60.

[50] Bowsher JG, Hussain A, Nevelos J, et al. The importance of head diameter in minimising metal-on-metal hip wear. In: Proceedings of the 50th Annual Meeting of the Orthopaedic Research Society. San Francisco, California. Rosemont (IL): Orthopaedic Research Society; 2004. p. 1453.

[51] Collins T, Carroll M, Timmerman I, et al. Wear of large diameter metal on metal hip bearings in primary and revision surface replacement. In: Transactions 50th Annual Meeting Orthopaedic Research Society, San Francisco, California. Rosemont (IL): Orthopaedic Research Society; 2004. p. 1452.

[52] Bowsher JG, Nevelos A, Pickard J, et al. Do heat treatments influence the wear of large diameter metal-on-metal hip joints? An in vitro study under normal and adverse gait conditions. In: Transactions 49th Annual Meeting Orthopaedic Research Society, New Orleans, Louisiana. Rosemont (IL): Orthopaedic Research Society; 2003. p. 1398.

[53] Dowling JM, Atkinson JR, Dowson D, et al. The characteristics of acetabular cups worn in the human body. J Bone Joint Surg [Br] 1978;60(3):375–82.

[54] Yamamoto K, Imakiire A, Shishido T, et al. Cementless total hip arthroplasty using porous-coated Biomet acetabular cups (Hexloc and Ringloc types). J Orthop Sci 2003;8(5):657–63.

[55] Eickmann T, Green DD, Donaldson T. Backside wear in retrieved hylamer liners. In: Brown S, Clarke IC, Gustafson A, editors. Proceedings of the 16th Annual Symposium of the International Society of Techniques in Arthroplasty. San Francisco, California, 2003. p. 172–5.

[56] Kothari M, Bartel DL, Booker JF. Surface geometry of retrieved McKee-Farrar total hip replacements. Clin Orthop 1996;329(Suppl):S141–7.

[57] Long WT, Dorr LD, Gendelman V. An American experience with metal-on-metal total hip arthroplasties: a 7-year follow-up study. J Arthroplasty 2004; 19(Suppl 3):29–34.

[58] Butterfield M, Stewart T, S. Williams, et al. Wear of metal-metal and ceramic-ceramic hip protheses with swing phase microseparation. In: Proceedings of the 48th Meeting of the Orthopaedic Research Society. Dallas, Texas. Rosemont (IL): Orthopaedic Research Society; 2002. p. 128.

[59] Griss P, Silber R, Merkle B, et al. Biomechanically induced tissue reactions after Al2O3-ceramic hip joint replacement. Experimental and early clinical results. J Biomed Mater Res 1976;10(4):519–28.

[60] Dorlot JM. Long-term effects of alumina components in total hip prostheses. Clin Orthop 1992;282:47–52.

[61] Manaka M, Clarke IC, Yamamoto K, et al. Stripe wear rates in alumina THR—comparison of micro-separation simulator study with retrieved implants. J Biomed Mater Res 2004;69B(2):149–57.

[62] Shishido T, Clarke IC, Williams P, et al. Clinical and simulator wear study of alumina ceramic THR to 17 years and beyond. J Biomed Mater Res 2003; 67B(1):638–47.

[63] McKellop HA, Campbell P, Park SH, et al. The origin of submicron polyethylene wear debris in total hip arthroplasty. Clin Orthop 1995;311:3–20.

[64] Furuya K, Tsuchiya M, Kawachi S. Socket-cup arthroplasty. Clin Orthop 1978;134:41–4.

[65] Furnes A, Lie SA, Havelin LI, et al. The economic impact of failures in total hip replacement surgery: 28,997 cases from the Norwegian Arthroplasty Register, 1987–1993. Acta Orthop Scand 1996;67(2): 115–21.

[66] Ohlin A. Failure of the Christiansen hip. Survival analysis of 265 cases. Acta Orthop Scand 1990;61(1): 7–11.

[67] Dennis DA, Komistek RD, Northcut EJ, et al. "In vivo" determination of hip joint separation and the forces generated due to impact loading conditions. J Biomech 2001;34(5):623–9.

[68] Iida H, Kaneda E, Takada H, et al. Metallosis due to impingement between the socket and the femoral neck in a metal-on-metal bearing total hip prosthesis. A case report. J Bone Joint Surg [Am] 1999;81(3): 400–3.

[69] Eickmann T, Manaka M, LC Clarke. Squeaking and neck-socket impingement in a ceramic total hip arthroplasty. In: Ben-Nissan B, Walsh W, Sher D, editors. Bioceramics-15, Sydney, Australia. Enfield (NH): Trans Tech Pub Ltd; 2002. p. 849–52.

[70] Willert HG, Buchhorn GH, Gobel D, et al. Wear behavior and histopathology of classic cemented metal on metal hip endoprostheses. Clin Orthop 1996; 329(Suppl):S160–86.

[71] Lhotka C, Szekeres T, Steffan I, et al. Four-year study of cobalt and chromium blood levels in patients managed with two different metal-on-metal total hip replacements. J Orthop Res 2003;21(2): 189–95.

[72] Campbell P, Shen FW, McKellop H. Biologic and tribologic considerations of alternative bearing surfaces. Clin Orthop 2004;418:98–111.

[73] Boehler N. Experiences with metal on metal components in THR. Acta Orthop Belg 1997;63(Suppl 1): 96–7.

[74] Doorn PF, Campbell PA, Worrall J, et al. Metal wear particle characterization from metal on metal total hip replacements: transmission electron microscopy study of periprosthetic tissues and isolated particles. J Biomed Mater Res 1998;42(1):103–11.

[75] MacDonald SJ, Brodner W, Jacobs JJ. A consensus paper on metal ions in metal-on-metal hip arthroplasties. J Arthroplasty 2004;19(8 Suppl 3):12–6.

[76] Campbell PA, Wang M, Amstutz HC, et al. Positive cytokine production in failed metal-on-metal total hip replacements. Acta Orthop Scand 2002;73(5):506–12.

[77] Jin ZM. Analysis of mixed lubrication mechanism in metal-on-metal hip joint replacements. Proc Inst Mech Eng [H] 2002;216(1):85–9.

[78] Skipor AK, Campbell PA, Patterson LM, et al. Serum and urine metal levels in patients with metal-on-metal surface arthroplasty. J Mater Sci Mater Med 2002; 13(12):1227–34.

[79] Takahashi T, Kuiper JH, Gile S, et al. Effect of exercise on metal levels in patients with three different metal-on-metal hip replacements. In: Proceedings of the American Academy of Orthopaedic Surgeons. San Francisco, California. American Academy of Orthopaedic Surgeons; 2004. p. 71.

[80] Beaule PE, Amstutz HC, Le Duff M, et al. Surface arthroplasty for osteonecrosis of the hip: hemiresurfacing versus metal-on-metal hybrid resurfacing. J Arthroplasty 2004;19(Suppl 3):54–8.

[81] Kim SY, Kyung HS, Ihn JC, et al. Cementless Metasul metal-on-metal total hip arthroplasty in patients less than fifty years old. J Bone Joint Surg [Am] 2004;86(11):2475–81.

[82] Brodner W, Grubl A, Jankovsky R, et al. Cup inclination and serum concentration of cobalt and chromium after metal-on-metal total hip arthroplasty. J Arthroplasty 2004;19(Suppl 3):66–70.

[83] Glyn-Jones S, Gill HS, McLardy-Smith P, et al. Roentgen stereophotogram-metric analysis of the Birmingham hip resurfacing arthroplasty. A two-year study. J Bone Joint Surg [Br] 2004;86(2):172–6.

[84] Hedley A, Moreland JR, Bloebaum R, et al. Press-fit, cemented, and bone ingrowth surface replacement—canine fixation model. In: Proceedings of the Annual Meeting of the Orthopaedic Research Society. San Francisco, California. Rosemont (IL): Orthopaedic Research Society; 1979. p. 163.

[85] Hedley A, Clarke IC, Bloebaum R, et al. Durability of acrylic cement fixation of femoral head prostheses—a canine surface replacement model. The Hip. Proceedings of the Hip Society. St. Louis: C.V. Mosby; 1979. p. 160.

[86] Reinisch G, Judmann KP, Lhotka C, et al. Retrieval study of uncemented metal-metal hip prostheses revised for early loosening. Biomaterials 2003;24(6): 1081–91.

[87] Al-Saffar N. Early clinical failure of total joint replacement in association with follicular prolifera-tion of B-lymphocytes: a report of two cases. J Bone Joint Surg [Am] 2002;84(12):2270–3.

[88] Urban RM, Jacobs JJ, Tomlinson MJ, et al. Dissemination of wear particles to the liver, spleen, and abdominal lymph nodes of patients with hip or knee replacement. J Bone Joint Surg [Am] 2000;82(4): 457–76.

[89] Case CP, Langkamer VG, James C, et al. Widespread dissemination of metal debris from implants. J Bone Joint Surg [Br] 1994;76(5):701–12.

[90] Jacobs JJ, Hallab NJ, Skipor AK, et al. Metal degradation products: a cause for concern in metal-metal bearings? Clin Orthop 2003;417:139–47.

[91] Weber BG. Experience with the Metasul total hip bearing system. Clin Orthop 1996;329(Suppl):S69–77.

[92] Hallab NJ, Anderson S, Caicedo M, et al. Immune responses correlate with serum-metal in metal-on-metal hip arthroplasty. J Arthroplasty 2004; 19(8 Suppl 3):88–93.

[93] Smith SL, Dowson D, Goldsmith AA. The effect of femoral head diameter upon lubrication and wear of metal-on-metal total hip replacements. Proc Inst Mech Eng [H] 2001;215(2):161–70.

[94] Clarke IC, Good V, Williams P, et al. Ultra-low wear rates for rigid-on-rigid bearings in total hip replacements. Proc Inst Mech Eng [H] 2000;214(4):331–47.

[95] Jacobs JJ, Skipor AK, Campbell PA, et al. Can metal levels be used to monitor metal-on-metal hip arthroplasties? J Arthroplasty 2004;19(8 Suppl 3):59–65.

[96] Lhotka C, Szekeres T, Steffan I, et al. Four-year study of cobalt and chromium blood levels in patients managed with two different metal-on-metal total hip replacements. J Orthop Res 2003;21(2):189–95.

[97] Lu B, Marti A, McKellop H. Wear of a second-generation metal-on-metal hip replacement effect of third-body abrasive particles. In: Transactions Sixth World Biomaterials Congress, Kamuela, Hawaii; 2000. p. 183.

[98] Walters Jr WL, Insley GM, Walter WK, et al. Edge loading in third generation alumina ceramic-on-ceramic bearings: Stripe wear. Presented at the Annual Meeting of American Academy of Orthopaedic Surgeons, February 2003, AAOS# 278.

[99] Walker PS, Salvati E, Hotzler RK. The wear on removed McKee-Farrar total hip prostheses. J Bone Joint Surg [Am] 1974;56:92–100.

ELSEVIER
SAUNDERS

Orthop Clin N Am 36 (2005) 163 – 170

ORTHOPEDIC
CLINICS
OF NORTH AMERICA

Anatomic Considerations for the Choice of Surgical Approach for Hip Resurfacing Arthroplasty

Sean E. Nork, MD, Michael Schär, Gilles Pfander, Martin Beck, MD,
Valentin Djonov, MD, Reinhold Ganz, MD, Michael Leunig, MD*

Department of Orthopaedic Surgery, University of Berne, Inselspital, CH-3010 Berne, Switzerland

In the first "Symposium on Surface Replacement Arthroplasty of the Hip" more than 2 decades ago, Harty [1] and Stulberg [2] suggested the vital role of maintaining the medial femoral circumflex artery (MFCA) in joint-preserving procedures such as hip resurfacing arthroplasty (HRA). In addition to this biologic consideration, Stulberg [2] advised that a sufficient surgical exposure is necessary to precisely prepare the acetabulum and the femur for accurate component positioning. On the femoral side, the pathologies that need to be addressed during HRA frequently include cysts, necrotic areas, postslip morphologies, and femoral neck abnormalities. These pathologies are almost exclusively located anteriorly, not posteriorly. Therefore, an anatmcially sound approach should allow proper visualization of deformities and correct placement of the components while minimizing the disruption to the soft tissues.

An anterior approach for HRA [3] requires a significantly larger soft tissue release compared with the approaches currently used for minimally invasive total hip arthroplasty. Even with a more extensive anterior approach, acetabular visualization remains difficult, and a potentially dangerous incision of the posterior capsule for its release may be necessary, putting the MFCA at risk. Alternatively, posterior approaches—advocated by many surgeons for total hip arthroplasty and frequently used in HRA— provide excellent exposure of the acetabulum and

the posterior femur. To obtain adequate exposure, however, all of the posterior muscles (from the piriformis to the tendinous insertion of the gluteus maximus) frequently require transection, which can be detrimental to the MFCA. Based on the authors' experience with intracapsular, hip-preserving procedures spanning more than 10 years, the most biologically respectful approach that facilitates an optimal exposure of the entire acetabulum and the femur is the technique of anterior surgical hip dislocation using a posterolateral transtrochanteric approach, which has previously been described for HRA [4].

To avoid unnecessary iatrogenic morbidity related to the lateral and posterolateral approaches, a detailed understanding of the topographic and surgical anatomy of the relevant structures is important. Although there are several publications describing the location of the superior gluteal nerve (SGN) at the proximal extent of the gluteus medius split in a transgluteal approach, to the authors' knowledge, there is minimal literature further detailing this subject [5–16]. For the gluteus maximus split in a classic Kocher-Langenbeck approach and the Gibson approach, the available literature is even scarcer. Finally, literature on surgical anatomy of the piriformis muscle and its relationship to the ascending branch of the MCFA is largely anecdotal. The purposes of this anatomic study are to (1) describe the locations of the inferior gluteal nerve (IGN) and inferior gluteal artery (IGA) and the SGN and superior gluteal artery (SGA) as they relate to the maximus muscle split of a Kocher-Langenbeck approach [17,18] or the maximus release of a Gibson [19] approach; (2) describe the relative

---

* Corresponding author.

  E-mail address: michael.leunig@balgrist.ch
(M. Leunig).

orthopedic.theclinics.com

locations of the inferior branch of the SGN and SGA as they relate to a transgluteal (Hardinge) approach [20]; and (3) further describe the anatomy of the piriformis muscle and its relation to vascular structures.

Materials and methods

The topographic anatomy of the neurovascular supply to the gluteus maximus and medius muscles were studied in 9 cadaver specimens; the topographic anatomy of the piriformis muscle was studied in an additional 14 cadaver specimens. All specimens were fixed in formaldehyde and ranged in age from 20 to 90 years.

The surgical approaches (Kocher-Langenbeck [17,18], Gibson [19], and Hardinge [20]) were defined before the anatomic dissections. Each dissection included identification of the relevant neurovascular structures as they related to each of these exposures. The following parameters were measured: the location of the anterior border of the gluteus maximus origin relative to the anterior superior iliac spine, the maximum length and width of the gluteus maximus muscle and tendon, the distance of the tendon to the lesser trochanter, and the course of the IGN. For the gluteus medius muscle, the maximum length and width, the location of the neurovascular pedicle as it exits the greater sciatic notch, the number and relative locations of the neurovascular structures supplying the gluteus maximus and medius, and the distance between the tip of the greater trochanter and the neurovascular structures were measured. For the piriformis muscle, the length and width of the muscular and tendinous portions of the muscle and its relation to nearby vascular structures were recorded.

The skin and subcutaneous tissues were removed from the lateral and posterior aspects of the hip and buttocks. The anterior border of the gluteus maximus was first defined and then dissected in a fashion similar to the Gibson approach. The gluteus maximus osseous insertion at the femur was incised, allowing partial mobilization from the underlying gluteus medius muscle belly. The shared fascia between the gluteus maximus and medius was mobilized with the maximus, maintaining the integrity of the neurovascular structures supplying the gluteus maximus. The gluteus medius origin from the iliac crest was then incised (with the tensor facsia lata muscle), allowing distal mobilization from the underlying minimus muscle. This facilitated exposure of the branches from the IGN/IGA and the SGN/SGA. Finally, the piriformis muscle belly and its tendinous

insertion were dissected from the gluteus medius and minimus muscles, allowing for precise measurements of its overall and muscle and tendon lengths. All dimensions were measured directly from the preparations and photographic documentation was used for most cases. Measurements are reported in centimeters as the mean plus or minus standard deviation with the range (minimum and maximum).

Anatomic approaches used

Kocher-Langenbeck gluteus maximus split
The gluteus maximus muscle was split in line with the fibers, in the direction of a line extending from the tip of the trochanter to the palpable posterior superior iliac spine as originally described by von Langenbeck [18] and later modified by Kocher [17].

Gibson release of gluteus maximus.   The anterior border of the gluteus maximus muscle was defined and dissected from its anterior insertion along the iliotibial band. Distally, the iliotibial band was incised in line with the midlateral aspect of the proximal femoral shaft.

Hardinge gluteus medius split.   For the transgluteal approach, there is significant variability in the described locations for initiation of the gluteus muscle split at the proximal aspect of the greater trochanter. Similar to that location described by Hardinge [20], we initiated the medius split at the palpable indentation of the anterior contour of the greater trochanter. This location leaves the posterior portion of the medius tendon insertion at the trochanteric tip intact and allows distal extension in the vastus lateral if necessary. This location optimizes protection of the gluteus medius muscle fibers posterior to the split during preparation of the femoral canal for total hip replacement.

Results

The Gibson release of the gluteus maximus from the iliotibial band is easily found by identifying the small blood vessels that perforate the iliotibial band at the anterior border of the gluteus maximus. The IGN and IGA branches were consistently located superficial to the shared fascia between the gluteus maximus and the medius muscles. To protect and maintain the integrity of these structures, this shared fascial layer required dissection and mobilization with the reflected maximus muscle belly. In the gluteus maximus splitting portion of the Kocher-

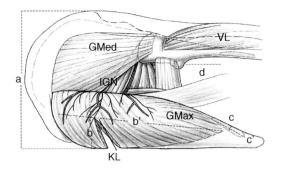

Fig. 1. The relationship between the gluteus maximus muscle (GMax) and the IGN during the Kocher-Langenbeck (KL) surgical approach. See Table 1 for measurements of a, b, b', c, c', and d. (GMed, gluteus medius muscle; VL, vastus lateralis muscle.)

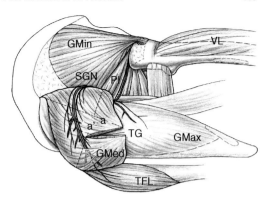

Fig. 2. The relationship between the gluteus medius muscle (GMed) and the inferior branch of the SGN in the transgluteal (TG) surgical approach. See Table 2 for measurements of a and a'. (GMax, gluteus maximus muscle; GMin, gluteus minimus muscle; PI, piriformis muscle; TFL, tensor fascia lata muscle; VL, vastus lateralis muscle.)

Langenbeck surgical approach (Fig. 1 and Table 1), the average distance between the greater trochanter and the first crossing neurovascular branch of the IGN/IGA was 8.7 cm (± 1.5 cm). In four of seven specimens, the artery was located inferior to the nerve. There was an average of 2.2 major neurovascular branches (range, 1–4) traveling along the undersurface of the maximus.

In the Hardinge-type gluteal splitting approach (Fig. 2 and Table 2), the average distance between the greater trochanter and the most distal branch of the SGN was 5.9 cm (± 1.1 cm), whereas the average distance to the SGA was 6.2 cm (± 0.9 cm). In six of eight specimens, the artery was located inferior to the nerve branch (ie, closer to the greater trochanter). The average distance between the artery and nerve was 4.7 mm. The SGN was noted to have an average of 2.4 major branches (range, 2–4). The primary branches of the SGN and SGA were located in a mobile tissue layer between the gluteus medius and minimus muscles, with branches supplying the

Table 1

Measurements of gluteus maximus muscle obtained from nine cadaveric specimens

Distance	Mean ± SD (cm)	Range (cm)
ASIS–anterior border of Gmax (a)	21.5 ± 2.4	18.0–24.5
GMax		
Width (b)	16.2 ± 1.8	16.0–18.0
Length (b')	27.1 ± 1.3	24.5–29.0
GMax tendon		
Width (c)	1.5 ± 0.4	0.9–2.4
Length (c')	5.7 ± 1.4	3.5–7.5
Lesser trochanter–GMax tendon (d)	2.0 ± 0.9	0.8–3.8
Anterior margin GMax–IGN (IGN) (1 branch 2 of 9, 2 branches 4 of 9, 3 branches 2 of 9, and 4 branches 1 of 9)	4.9 ± 1.7	0.3–7.3
Kocher-Langenbeck incision–IGN (KL)		
Nerve	8.7 ± 1.5	4.8–13.2
Artery	8.7 ± 0.6	7.8–10.2

Abbreviations: ASIS, anterior superior iliac spine; GMax, gluteus maximus muscle; KL, Kocher-Langenbeck.

Table 2

Measurements of gluteus medius muscle obtained from nine cadaveric specimens

Distance	Mean ± SD (cm)	Range (cm)
GMed		
Width (a)	13.6 ± 1.9	11.0–18.0
Length (a')	17.9 ± 1.8	14.5–20.5
Anterior margin GMed–SGN (SGN) (1 branch 0 of 9, 2 branches 6 of 9, 3 branches 2 of 9, and 4 branches 1 of 9)	3.8 ± 1.7	1.2–7.1
Transgluteal GMed split–SGN (TG)		
Nerve	5.9 ± 1.1	4.2–9.0
Artery	6.2 ± 0.9	4.8 ± 8.5

Abbreviations: GMed, gluteus medius muscle; TG, transgluteal gluteus medius split.

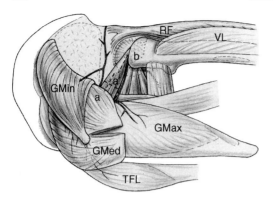

Fig. 3. The piriformis muscle is an important landmark for the course of the acetabular branch of the SGA and the anastomosis of the IGA with the MFCA. See Table 3 for measurements of a, a′, and b. (GMax, gluteus maximus muscle; GMed, gluteus medius muscle; GMin, gluteus minimus muscle; RF, rectus femoris muscle; TFL, tensor fascia lata muscle; VL, vastus lateralis muscle.)

muscles at numerous locations along their lengths. On average, the SGN entered the gluteus medius 3.8 cm (± 1.7 cm) proximal to the tensor fascia lata muscle. In one cadaver, branches of the SGN entered the tensor fascia lata muscle directly.

In all cases, the pirformis muscle inserted at the anterior half of the tip of the greater trochanter (Fig. 3 and Table 3). The length of the muscular portion of the piriformis was 6.4 cm (± 1.2 cm) with a diameter of 2.9 cm (± 0.7 cm). Superficially, the tendon length was 5.0 cm (± 0.7 cm). The deep portion of the tendon blended into the muscular piriformis and measured 7.5 cm (± 0.7 cm). In all cases, a branch of the IGA was found at the inferior border of the piriformis muscle (an anastomosis with the MFCA). At the superior border of the muscular portion of the piriformis muscle, the acetabular branch of the SGA was identified in all cases.

Discussion

With the renewed interest in bone-preserving procedures such as HRA, the question again arises: What role does the choice of surgical approach have on the clinical outcome? In a routine total hip arthroplasty, most of the reconstruction is built into the prosthetic design itself. In contrast, reconstruction with HRA is more dependent on preservation of the local biology of the acetabulum and proximal femur.

An insufficient appreciation of soft tissue anatomy may be associated with compromised patient outcomes and may lead to the inaccurate interpretation of surgical morbidity as an uncontrollable accident. Frequently, the operative details of a particular surgical approach are obtained from textbooks, some of which have been formulated decades ago and transcribed from edition to edition without substantive changes. These surgical approaches frequently use the principle of approaching the bone in the most direct way, assuming minimal risk and injury to the local nerves and vessels. An illustrative example of how this can negatively influence hip surgery and has slowed progress in hip joint–preserving procedures is the classic misunderstanding of femoral head blood supply preservation. Numerous textbooks have recommended ligation of the MFCA and its anastamoses [21–23], a clear attack on the perfusion of the femoral head [1,24–26]. More recent anatomic and clinical research has demonstrated (Fig. 4) that it is possible to perform intracapsular hip procedures and safely perform surgical dislocation without causing osteonecrosis [27].

Table 3
Measurements of piriformis muscle obtained from 14 cadaveric specimens

Distance	Mean ± SD (cm)	Range (cm)
Muscle dimensions		
Length (a)	6.4 ± 1.2	3.3–8.1
Diameter (a′)	2.9 ± 0.7	0.9–4.8
Tendon length		
Superficial (b)	5.0 ± 0.7	3.5–6.5
Deep	7.5 ± 0.7	6.5–10.5

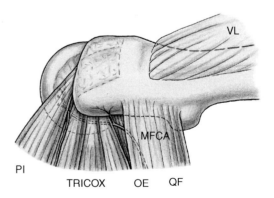

Fig. 4. The relevant deep anatomic structures of the posterior aspect of the hip, emphasizing the course of the MFCA to the femoral head. (OE, obturator externus muscle; QF, quadratus femoris muscle; PI, piriformis muscle; TRICOX, triceps coxae muscle; VL, vastus lateralis muscle.)

Although the introduction of metal-on-metal bearings may minimize wear-related failures, optimal implant fixation remains the key to a successful arthroplasty [28]. In that respect, impairment or compromise of the blood supply to the femoral head or neck during HRA as a result of surgical trauma or femoral head preparation could cause a sufficiently large necrotic fragment, endangering fixation of the femoral component or even leading to fracture of the femoral neck. The potential impact of impaired femoral head blood supply is especially relevant as cementless fixation of the femoral component and designs that minimize femoral head resection are considered. One possible reason why necrosis of the bone covered by the prosthesis is so rare is that current HRA procedures are epiphyseal resection arthroplasties and not true head resurfacing arthroplasties.

Kocher-Langenbeck and Gibson

The location of the IGN/IGA between the gluteus maximus and medius has implications for the Kocher-Langenbeck and the Gibson surgical exposures. In a maximus splitting exposure (Kocher-Langenbeck), dissection of the deep fascia shared by the gluteus maximus and medius (Fig. 5) should be limited based on the neurovascular anatomic location. The location of the most distal crossing gluteal nerve branch from the greater trochanter was variable in this study but was identified at a minimum distance of 7 cm. The anatomic proximity of these two neurovascular structures suggests the potential for nerve damage during hemostasis. Intraoperatively, vigorous

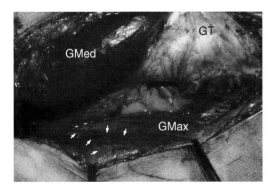

Fig. 5. Intraoperative photograph of the surgical exposure using a Gibson approach with release of the gluteus maximus muscle (GMax) from the iliotibial band. The arrows indicate the blood vessels located in the interfascial layer between the maximus and medius muscles, which should stay with the GMax to preserve its neurovascular supply. (GMed, gluteus medius muscle; GT, greater trochanter.)

bleeding from the gluteus maximus may be indicative of direct IGN damage because the IGN and vessels travel along an almost identical course. Intraoperatively, this close relationship is evidenced by the frequently observed massive muscle contraction that occurs with electrocautery in this area, indicative of the close proximity of the nerve and vessel. The location of these branches in the shared fascia between the maximus and medius muscles suggests that an anterior, maximus-sparing approach (Gibson) should include dissection of the shared fascia strictly with the maximus. The preservation of the shared fascia in the Gibson approach ensures maintenance of the neurovascular supply to the maximus and avoids the potential damage induced by the maximus split.

The gluteus maximus functions as a powerful hip extensor [29]. Local fibrosis or weakness likely has a negative affect on hip function, especially in the young and active patient; however, the literature on the effects of an islolated insufficiency of the gluteus maximus muscle is scarce. Although the gluteus maximus has been used as a soft tissue transfer for local pressure sores and anorectal soft tissue defects [30], the clinically relevant effects are unknown. Presumably, maximizing the function of the gluteus maximus by respecting its innervation during a surgical approach for HRA should optimize outcomes and hip function.

Hardinge

Using the midportion of the greater trochanter as a reference point, the branches of the SGA/SGN were located as close as 4 cm cephalad. Alternatively stated, splitting the medius beyond 4 cm at the midportion of the greater trochanter places the inferior branch of the SGN at risk. Similar to the IGN/IGA, the SGN coursed parallel and adjacent to the inferior branch of the SGA (mean distance between the artery and nerve was 4.7 mm), and in 75% of specimens, the artery was caudal to the nerve. As a result, the presence of vigorous bleeding intraoperatively at the proximal extension of the gluteus medius split is likely indicative of a nerve injury, given the usual location of the vessel caudad to the inferior branch of the SGN. In addition, the use of electrocautery during hemostasis may image the inferior branch of the SGN.

Although information on the neurovasculature of the gluteus maximus is scarce, the relative location of the inferior branch of the SGN with respect to the gluteus medius muscle has been emphasized in numerous previous publications and anatomic studies. Although significant variation exists in the "safe area" [5–16] for cephalad dissection, most investigators have reported a safe distance of 5 cm relative to the greater trochanter. The maximum distance of the split from the greater trochanter, however, depends on additional factors including the size of the patient and the anatomic location of the split itself relative to the tip of the greater trochanter [7,12, 14,15]. The inferior branch of the SGN has been shown to course obliquely form cephalad to caudad (ie, closer to the greater trochanter) as the nerve travels from posterior to anterior [12,14]. Injury to the branches of the SGN during transgluteal approaches has been described in numerous reports [5,7,9,10,13, 31,32], resulting in weakness of the gluteus medius or tensor fascia (or both). This weakness can be associated with significant functional limitations, most notably a Trendelenburg gait [5,9,16,31,32]. Reported persistence of electromyogram-confirmed abductor muscle dysfunction after hip arthroplasty through a lateral approach has ranged from 8% to 40%; however, the incidence of clinically significant muscle dysfunction is observed less commonly [5,7,31,32]. It is postulated that the main branch of the nerve (which is embedded between in the interfascial layer between the gluteus medius and minimus) may be able to escape some degree of blunt trauma.

Piriformis muscle

The piriformis muscle parallels the posterior margin of the gluteus medius and minimus muscles. It originates from second to the fourth sacral vertebral body. The muscle runs through the greater sciatic notch and is attached by a round tendon to the upper border of the greater trochanter anterosuperior to the trochanteric fossa, where it is cushioned by a bursa. At the inferior margin of the piriformis, the final anastomosis between the MFCA and the IGA is located. At the superior margin of the piriformis, the superior acetabular branch of the SGA is located. The piriformis therefore represents an important anatomic landmark: safe surgical dissection to the hip capsule should be proximal to this structure.

Literature regarding the piriformis muscle has mainly focused on the piriformis syndrome and the anomalous relationship between the sciatic nerve and the piriformis [33]; its anatomic relationships have been reported on less frequently [34]. In particular, the importance of this muscle as an anatomic landmark has not been emphasized. Assuming the importance of the MFCA for femoral head viability, dissections caudal to the piriformis tendon must be avoided.

The location of the piriformis insertion was in the middle of the upper border of the greater trochanter and expanded up to its anterosuperior peak, which is in contradistinction to the presumed locations at the posterosuperior trochanter or even in the piriformis fossa. These anatomic nuances are useful for the transgluteal approach because the piriformis tendon is easily traceable and can serve as a point of orientation. By remaining cephalad to the piriformis, the gluteus minimus muscles can be released from the hip joint capsule without laceration of their fibers, which may be especially important in minimizing the formation of ectopic bone during surgical exposures in this region. Finally, the variable length of the piriformis tendon observed may be of clinical interest, explaining the commonly observed difference in elasticty noted during surgical dissection.

Summary

With respect to soft tissue preservation during lateral and posterolateral approaches, the following may be advisable based on the anatomic observations of this study.

1. To maximize the surgical exposure while minimizing damage to the associated neurovascular structures, the gluteus maximus should be released from its anterior insertion at the iliotibial band (as in the Gibson approach) rather than split (as in the Kocher-Langenbeck approach). This method is recommended because of the high variability in the course of the IGN/IGA structures that may be located as close as 7 cm to the greater trochanter. The shared fascial layer between the gluteus maximus and medius should be maintained with the maximus during the Gibson approach, ensuring the integrity of the neurovascular branches that supply the maximus muscle.
2. For the transgluteal (Hardinge) approach, the proximal extension of the gluteus medius muscle split should be limited to 4 to 5 cm from the tip of the greater trochanter. This muscle split should be even shorter at the anterior trochanter. This anatomic limitation suggests that a surgical dislocation (for intracapsular procedures, HRA, femoral neck osteotomy, or other procedures) performed through a gluteus medius splitting approach is limited by the size of the femoral head and neck. Given the relative anatomic size of these structures, neurovascular damage to the SGA is likely.

3. The piriformis muscle is a posterior hip stabilizer and its tendon inserts at the tip of the greater trochanter. It is a landmark for the identification of the anastomosis with the MFCA. The deep branch of the MFCA is located distal to the piriformis and it perforates the hip capsule in this location. Therefore, approaching the hip from posterior endangers this vessel, in particular, if the posterior approach extends distally to the piriformis tendon. The dislocation of the hip anterior or posterior is not critical so long as the obturator externus tendon is intact (protector of MCFA); however, the execution of a posterior approach to allow sufficient mobilization of the proximal femur includes the release of the short external rotators, including the obturator externus.

4. Finally, based on the authors' anatomic dissections and the capacity of preserving femoral head vascularity during intracapsular procedures of the hip such as HRA, the digastric trochanteric osteotomy (also known as the trochanteric slide osteotomy) is ideally suited to providing optimal exposure of the acetabulum and the proximal femur and maintaining the soft tissue integrity of the hip joint. As such, it facilitates the correction of proximal femoral abnormalities of the head ("pistol grip") or neck (short, varus) that need to be addressed to obtain a sufficient intra- and extra-articular hip clearance.

References

[1] Harty M. Symposium on Surface Replacement Arthroplasty of the Hip. Anatomic considerations. Orthop Clin N Am 1982;13(4):667–79.

[2] Stulberg SD. Surgical approaches for the performance of surface replacement arthroplasties. Orthop Clin N Am 1982;13(4):739–46.

[3] Wagner H. Surface replacement arthroplasty of the hip. Clin Orthop 1978;134:102–30.

[4] Beaule PE. A soft tissue-sparing approach to surface arthroplasty of the hip. Oper Tech Ortho 2004;14(2):75–84.

[5] Abitbol JJ, Gendron D, Laurin CA, et al. Gluteal nerve damage following total hip arthroplasty. A prospective analysis. J Arthroplasty 1990;5(4):319–22.

[6] Akita K, Sakamoto H, Sato T. Origin, course and distribution of the superior gluteal nerve. Acta Anat (Basel) 1994;149(3):225–30.

[7] Baker AS, Bitounis VC. Abductor function after total hip replacement. An electromyographic and clinical review. J Bone Joint Surg Br 1989;71(1):47–50.

[8] Bos JC, Stoeckart R, Klooswijk AI, et al. The surgical anatomy of the superior gluteal nerve and anatomical radiologic bases of the direct lateral approach to the hip. Surg Radiol Anat 1994;16(3):253–8.

[9] Comstock C, Imrie S, Goodman SB. A clinical and radiographic study of the "safe area" using the direct lateral approach for total hip arthroplasty. J Arthroplasty 1994;9(5):527–31.

[10] Dall D. Exposure of the hip by anterior osteotomy of the greater trochanter. A modified anterolateral approach. J Bone Joint Surg Br 1986;68(3):382–6.

[11] Duparc F, Thomine JM, Dujardin F, et al. Anatomic basis of the transgluteal approach to the hip-joint by anterior hemimyotomy of the gluteus medius. Surg Radiol Anat 1997;19(2):61–7.

[12] Eksioglu F, Uslu M, Gudemez E, et al. Reliability of the safe area for the superior gluteal nerve. Clin Orthop 2003;412:111–6.

[13] Frndak PA, Mallory TH, Lombardi Jr AV. Translateral surgical approach to the hip. The abductor muscle "split." Clin Orthop 1993;295:135–41.

[14] Jacobs LG, Buxton RA. The course of the superior gluteal nerve in the lateral approach to the hip. J Bone Joint Surg Am 1989;71(8):1239–43.

[15] Lavigne P, Loriot de Rouvray TH. [The superior gluteal nerve. Anatomical study of its extrapelvic portion and surgical resolution by trans-gluteal approach]. Rev Chir Orthop Reparatrice Appar Mot 1994;80(3):188–95.

[16] Nazarian S, Tisserand P, Brunet C, et al. Anatomic basis of the transgluteal approach to the hip. Surg Radiol Anat 1987;9(1):27–35.

[17] Kocher T. Chirurgische operationslehre, vol. 5. 5th edition. Jena, Germany: Gustav Fischer; 1907.

[18] von Langenbeck B. Ueber Schussverletzungen des Hüftgelenks. Arch Klin Chirurg 1874;16:263.

[19] Gibson A. A posterior exposure of the hip. J Bone Joint Surg Br 1950;32:183–6.

[20] Hardinge K. The direct lateral approach to the hip. J Bone Joint Surg Br 1982;64(1):17–9.

[21] Hastings DE, Sullivan JM, Colton CL. The hip. In: Colton CL, Hall AJ, editors. Atlas of Orthopaedic Surgical Approaches. Oxford (UK): Butterworth-Heinemann; 1991. p. 1–23.

[22] Zinghi GF, et al. Le fratture della pelvi e del cotile, vol. 1. Bologna, Italy: Timeo; 2000. p. 133–50.

[23] Rüedi T, von Hochstetter AHC, Schlumpf R. Operative Zugänge der Osteosynthese, vol. 1. New York: Thieme; 1984. p. 101–8.

[24] Gautier E, et al. Anatomy of the medial femoral circumflex artery and its surgical implications. J Bone Joint Surg Br 2000;82(5):679–83.

[25] Ogden JA. Changing patterns of proximal femoral vascularity. J Bone Joint Surg Am 1974;56(5):941–50.

[26] Sevitt S, Thompson RG. The distribution and anastomoses of arteries supplying the head and neck of the femur. J Bone Joint Surg Br 1965;47(3):560–73.

[27] Ganz R, Gill TJ, Gautier E, et al. Surgical dislocation of the adult hip a technique with full access to the

femoral head and acetabulum without the risk of avascular necrosis. J Bone Joint Surg Br 2001;83(8): 1119–24.

[28] Beaule PE, Le Duff M, Campbell P, et al. Metal-on-metal surface arthroplasty with a cemented femoral component: a 7–10 year follow-up study. J Arthroplasty 2004;19(8 Suppl 3):17–22.

[29] van der Linden ML, Hazlewood ME, Aitchison AM, et al. Electrical stimulation of gluteus maximus in children with cerebral palsy: effects on gait characteristics and muscle strength. Dev Med Child Neurol 2003;45(6):385–90.

[30] Christiansen J, Hansen CR, Rasmussen O. Bilateral gluteus maximus transposition for anal incontinence. Br J Surg 1995;82(7):903–5.

[31] Siebenrock KA, Rosler KM, Gonzalez E, et al. Intraoperative electromyography of the superior gluteal nerve during lateral approach to the hip for arthroplasty: a prospective study of 12 patients. J Arthroplasty 2000;15(7):867–70.

[32] Ramesh M, O'Byrne JM, McCarthy N, et al. Damage to the superior gluteal nerve after the Hardinge approach to the hip. J Bone Joint Surg Br 1996;78(6): 903–6.

[33] Parziale JR, Hudgins TH, Fishman LM. The piriformis syndrome. Am J Orthop 1996;25(12):819–23.

[34] Akita K, Sakamoto H, Sato T. Arrangement and innervation of the glutei medius and minimus and the piriformis: a morphological analysis. Anat Rec 1994; 238(1):125–30.

ELSEVIER
SAUNDERS

Orthop Clin N Am 36 (2005) 171 – 176

ORTHOPEDIC
CLINICS
OF NORTH AMERICA

Distribution of Vascular Foramina Around the Femoral Head and Neck Junction: Relevance for Conservative Intracapsular Procedures of the Hip

Martin Lavigne, MD, FRCSC, Morteza Kalhor, MD, Martin Beck, MD, Reinhold Ganz, MD, Michael Leunig, MD*

Department of Orthopaedic Surgery, University of Berne, Inselspital, CH-3010 Berne, Switzerland

The preservation of blood supply to the femoral head is critical during open or arthroscopic intracapsular surgical procedures of the hip for the treatment of prearthritic conditions [1] to avoid avascular necrosis of the femoral head [2,3]. In the case of resurfacing arthroplasty for advanced hip joint degeneration, however, there is still a debate concerning the importance of preserving the femoral head and neck blood supply to ensure long-term success of the procedure. The blood supply to the femoral head has been studied in the past, with emphasis on the critical role of the deep branch of the medial femoral circumflex artery (traveling under the short rotators) and the lateral retinacular vessels in children and adults [4–7]. The contributions of the inferior or anterior retinacular vessels, the foveolar vessels, or the anastomoses between the epiphyseal and metaphyseal vessels are negligible or absent in the normal adult femoral head [7–11].

Despite growing interest in joint-preserving procedures for the treatment of femoroacetabular impingement [12] and in femoral head resurfacing arthroplasty for the treatment of advanced hip-joint degeneration, the precise vascular anatomy of the femoral head and neck junction is not well defined. It has been demonstrated that the lateral retinacular vessels lie on the posterolateral femoral neck embedded in a synovial membrane and reach the femoral head through nutrient vascular foramina, but no quantitative information exists on the exact location and distribution of the retinacular vessels at the head and neck junction. This study was designed to quantitatively determine the topographic anatomy of the terminal course of the medial femoral circumflex artery (retinacular vessels) to avoid damage to the vessels during intracapsular surgical procedures.

Materials and methods

The authors analyzed 150 dried cadaver femora from the Department of Anatomy, University of Berne, Switzerland and from the Institute of Anthropology, Basel, Switzerland. These specimens, obtained through a voluntary donor program or found during excavation in different parts of Switzerland, were preserved for teaching purposes. Information on age, sex, pre-existence of hip disease, or cause of death was not available. Only nonarthritic femora with a closed epiphyseal growth plate were used for the study.

The amount and distribution of vascular foramina located at the head and neck junction were counted and documented photographically. The femoral head and neck junction was divided into 12 sectors corresponding to a clock system (Fig. 1). Twelve o'clock and 6 o'clock were defined as the most superior and inferior points of the femoral head (in

———————
* Corresponding author.
E-mail address: michael.leunig@balgrist.ch
(M. Leunig).

the axis of the femur); 9 o'clock and 3 o'clock were defined as the posterior and anterior pole of the femoral head, respectively. The head and neck junction was defined as an area that was within 10 mm distal to the edge of the former articular cartilage of the femoral head. Only foramina with a diameter greater than 0.5 mm were recorded. The vascular foramina were quantified directly from the femora by loupe magnification. For ease of data processing, right-side equivalents were calculated for all femora. From 150 femora available for the study, 59 had to be excluded because of damage to the head and neck junction, leaving 38 right and 53 left femora for analysis.

Results

The average number of vascular foramina recorded was 15 (range, 8–21) per femur. The distribution of the foramina according to the clock system is shown in Fig. 2. An average of 7.5 foramina was found on the posterior area of the lateral neck (9–12 o'clock), which accounted for 49% of all foramina, with 8.5%, 16.5%, and 24% located between 9 and 10, 10 and 11, and 11 and 12 o'clock, respectively. Thirty-two percent of all

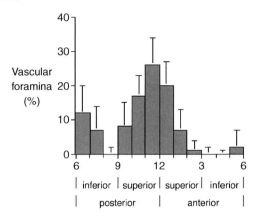

Fig. 2. Frequency distribution of vascular foramina. Foramina were most frequently observed (80%) at the antero- and posterosuperior regions of the femoral head neck junction. Anteriorly, only a few vascular foramina were identified.

foramina were located on the anterior area of the neck (12–6 o'clock), with most of them (88%) observed between 12 and 2 o'clock. Therefore, most of the foramina (77%) were located between 9 and 2 o'clock. Only a few foramina (4%) were found between 2 and 6 o'clock (see Fig. 2). No foramen was observed between 2 and 6 o'clock in 65 femora (71%). Another peak of foramina (19%) was located in the posteroinferior head and neck area (6–8 o'clock).

Discussion

Vascular foramina have been used to study the pattern of vascularization of specific bones such as the distal femur [13], vertebral bodies [14], the hook of hamate [15], the scaphoid [16], the incus [17], human long bones [18], and the navicular bone in horses [19]. For the same purpose, Jung et al [20] described the distribution of vascular foramina located at the femoral head and neck junction in 30 cadaver femora. From that study, however, it is difficult to draw precise conclusions because there is no information on the size of the foramina recorded or on the area defining the head and neck junction or their quadrant system. In the authors' study, most (77%) of vascular foramina were located between 9 and 2 o'clock, of which about one third (28%) were located between 12 and 2 o'clock (anterolateral area), whereas only 4% of all foramina were located between 2 and 6 o'clock. In 71% of the femora, the vascular foramina were completely missing from the

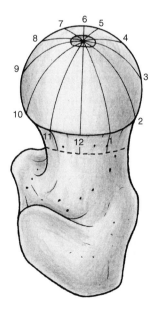

Fig. 1. The clock system used to represent the distribution of the vascular foramina. At the head and neck junction area (up to 10 mm from the articular cartilage), vascular foramina with a diameter of more than 0.5 mm were recorded.

anterior neck (2–6 o'clock). The paucity of vascular foramina identified at the anterior head and neck junction is in accordance with previous studies [5,7–10] and has been explained by the regression of these vessels as the neck grows [7]. Nevertheless, many vascular foramina were observed in proximity to the anterolateral area, and care should be taken when approaching this area along with the posterolateral area of the femoral head and neck junction during surgery.

The recorded foramina were clearly visible and of various sizes. The diameter of the retinacular arteries ranged from 0.10 to 1.55 mm in adults, with a mean diameter of 0.84 mm for the posterolateral retinacular vessels and 0.25 mm for the anterior retinacular vessels [9]. These diameter measurements do not take into account the loose connective tissue in which they are embedded and the corresponding venous plexus [21], which makes the necessary diameter of the corresponding foramen much larger. By recording foramina with a diameter as small as 0.5 mm, the number of vessels supplying blood to the femoral head was most likely overestimated. In addition, the authors considered the head and neck junction as a large area extending up to 10 mm distal to the edge of the former articular cartilage of the femoral head. In children, the retinacular vessels must pass over the physis to enter the femoral head [5,7]; in adults, this proximal entrance is maintained with the vessels penetrating the head at the articular rim. It is likely that some of the foramina recorded represent metaphyseal branches of the lateral retinacular vessels supplying blood to the femoral neck [22] or anasto-

moses between epiphyseal and metaphyseal branches of the lateral retinacular arteries [5]. The authors believe, however, that overestimating the number of foramina is prudent in light of the potential risk of avascular necrosis if the vessels are damaged.

Precise knowledge of vascular supply of the femoral head is important when considering surgical procedures around the femoral head and neck junction. This is true for open surgery that addresses the problem of impingement of the hip joint [12] and for arthroscopy-assisted osteoplasties of the hip. It is also important when surgical hip joint dislocation is performed for other indications [23–25].

Although Harty [21] suggested the potentially important role of the medial femoral circumflex artery for hip resurfacing more than 20 years ago, the importance of maintaining blood supply to the femoral head and neck during resurfacing arthroplasty of the hip joint in advanced hip disease is still being debated. Even though many surgeons use a posterior approach to the hip joint (which inevitably damages the deep branch of the medial femoral circumflex artery traveling under the short rotators, thus disrupting the main blood supply to the femoral head), most studies on hip resurfacing (hemi or total) have not reported femoral head necrosis as a significant problem [26,27]. This might be explained as follows: with current component designs and bone preparation techniques, most of the femoral head epiphysis is resected, producing a cylindric neck stump that includes only the posterolateral epiphysis onto which the femoral component is fitted (Fig. 3). This assumption may be confirmed by Bradley et al's

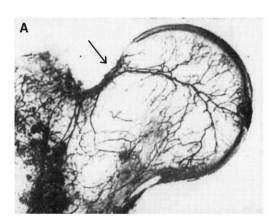
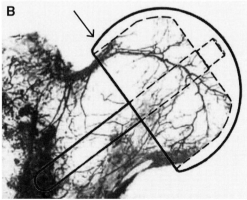

Fig. 3. Appearance of the femoral head epiphysis (part of the femoral head proximal to the large intraosseous vessel crossing the femoral head from lateral to medial) before (*A*) and after (*B*) insertion of the femoral component. Note that the large area of the epiphysis, which is perfused mainly by the lateral retinacular vessels (*arrow*), is resected after femoral head preparation. (*Adapted from* Sevitt S, Thompson RG. The distribution and anastomoses of arteries supplying the head and neck of the femur. J Bone Joint Surg [Br] 1965;47(3):563; with permission.)

[28] observation of bone necrosis that was located precisely in the posterolateral region of the resurfaced head under two failed femoral components, the remainder of the femoral head being still viable. It could be hypothesized that implant designs aimed at preserving more of the femoral head epiphysis may be at even greater risk of loosening/fracture because they rely more on the head than the neck.

Freeman [29] proposed, from his own observations, that most of the blood supply to the arthritic femoral head comes from intraosseous vessels instead of subsynovial vessels at the surface of the femoral neck. Studies in dog femoral heads tend to confirm the critical importance of the retinacular vessels in nonarthritic heads but also demonstrate evidence of significant collateral blood flow developing from the metaphysis in arthritic femoral heads [30–32]. This metaphyseal blood flow could explain the normal radionucleide uptake observed in the femoral head and neck after resurfacing arthroplasty [33]. A microvascular injection technique performed on the normal dog femoral head revealed the absence of blood flow after stripping the retinacular vessels [34], which is in accordance with studies in humans [6]. In the arthritic dog femoral head, blood flow was significantly decreased by as much as 75% (average, 50%) after combined stripping of the retinacular vessels and reaming of the head, suggesting the presence of only a few vascular anastomoses between the femoral epiphysis and metaphysis in some femoral heads. In the arthritic human femoral head, laser Doppler flow measurements demonstrate a sharp decline of as much as 90% in blood perfusion after stripping the retinacular vessels, confirming that intraosseous vascularization does not develop significantly in all patients (Schoeniger, personal communication, 2002). Beaulé et al [35] found a decrease in blood flow in the adult arthritic femoral head that varied from less than 5% to nearly 90% after intentional neck notching in patients undergoing total hip arthroplasty. Therefore, it seems that surgeons should not count on fully established "intraosseous neovascularization" from the metaphysis to compensate for the loss of blood supply from the retinacular vessels in all patients. The significance of intraosseous compensatory blood supply may depend on the preoperative diagnosis. It may also develop to some extent postoperatively in cases in which a relative ischemic situation is produced by the surgical procedure.

Some surgeons still believe that preserving blood supply to the resurfaced head and neck with the current technique of hip resurfacing is desirable, as was proposed early on by Harty [21]. Although not proved, preserving a more abundant blood supply could have a cooling effect when the femoral component is cemented, thus reducing the potential for heat-induced bone necrosis [26]. Moreover, bone remodeling and long-term fixation of an uncemented femoral component might be better achieved if good blood supply is available, although uncemented fixation for the femoral component has not yet demonstrated a specific mode of failure due to a lack of bone integration or remodeling. Finally, the delivery of antibiotics for prophylaxis or in case of proven infection may be improved with normal vascularization.

In a more biologic approach of femoral head resurfacing, the preservation of blood vessels is important. Femoral head viability is mandatory in procedures such as partial resurfacing of the femoral head [36], during "autogenous" resurfacing for osteonecrosis by the trap-door procedure [37], or in techniques involving resurfacing of a damaged femoral head with an allograft [38]. Femoral head viability will also be necessary in the future for procedures involving resurfacing with autologous chondrocytes transplantation. In addition, the preservation of optimal blood supply to the epiphysis would favor long-term fixation with a less aggressive form of resurfacing arthroplasty, using a smaller component design that replaces only the femoral head cartilage.

It is still possible with current resurfacing arthroplasty designs and techniques to protect the blood supply of the femoral head. Instead of using the more popular posterior approach, an anterior or transtrochanteric sliding osteotomy approach may be used [25]. A posterior approach with sectioning of the short rotators 1 cm from their insertion in the trochanteric crest, however, should protect the deep branch of the femoral circumflex artery, although this vessel would still be at risk from a stretch injury during dislocation of the joint and mobilization of the proximal femur [11]. Care should be taken to avoid damaging the retinacular vessels during circumferential capsulotomy, during preparation of the femoral head and neck with reamers, and when using centering stylus and retractors around the head and neck junction. Avoidance of high valgus positioning of the component or lateral neck notching lessens the risk of injury to the retinacular vessels [35]. Careful sizing of the component without removing too much bone from the femoral head and neck junction will effectively reproduce the anatomy and protect the vessels. Osteophyte resection should be performed with caution, especially in the postero- and anterolateral areas of the femoral neck.

Summary

Only a few vessels reach the adult femoral head on its anterior aspect, suggesting that surgical procedures on the anterior femoral head and neck can be safely performed by open and closed techniques (arthroscopy). Caution should be used, however, when approaching the anterolateral and posterolateral head and neck junction. The anatomic course of the deep branch of the medial circumflex artery should also be respected if a blood-sparing approach to femoral head resurfacing arthroplasty is contemplated, but it is still not known whether long-term survival of the femoral component is affected by the quality of the remaining femoral head and neck blood supply.

Acknowledgments

The authors thank B. Kaufmann from the Institute of Anthropology in Aesch, Switzerland and P. Eggli and V. Djonov from the Anatomical Institute, University of Berne, Switzerland for providing access to the femoral skeletons studied.

References

[1] Ganz R, Parvizi J, Beck M, et al. Femoroacetabular impingement: a cause for osteoarthritis of the hip. Clin Orthop 2003;417:112–20.

[2] Epstein H. Traumatic dislocations of the hip. Clin Orthop 1973;92:116–42.

[3] Epstein H. Posterior fracture-dislocations of the hip: long-term follow-up. J Bone Joint Surg Am 1974;56: 1103–27.

[4] Crock HV. An atlas of vascular anatomy of the skeleton and spinal cord. Martin Dunitz; 1996.

[5] Chung SMK. The arterial supply of the developing proximal end of the human femur. J Bone Joint Surg Am 1976;58(7):961–70.

[6] Notzli HP, Siebenrock KA, Hempfing A, et al. Perfusion of the femoral head during surgical dislocation of the hip. Monitoring by laser Doppler flowmetry. J Bone Joint Surg Br 2002;84(2):300–4.

[7] Ogden JA. Changing patterns of proximal femoral vascularity. J Bone Joint Surg Am 1974;56(5):941–50.

[8] Sevitt S, Thompson RG. The distribution and anastomoses of arteries supplying the head and neck of the femur. J Bone Joint Surg Br 1965;47(3):560–73.

[9] Tucker FR. Arterial supply of the femoral head and its clinical importance. J Bone Joint Surg Br 1949; 31(1):82–93.

[10] Howe WWJ, Lacey T, Schwartz P. A study of the gross anatomy of the arteries supplying the proximal portion of the femur and the acetabulum. J Bone Joint Surg Am 1950;32(4):856–66.

[11] Gautier E, Ganz K, Krugel N, et al. Anatomy of the medial femoral circumflex artery and its surgical implications. J Bone Joint Surg Br 2000;82(5):679–83.

[12] Lavigne M, Parvizi J, Beck M, et al. Anterior femoroacetabular impingement: part I. Techniques of joint preserving surgery. Clin Orthop 2004;418:61–6.

[13] Rogers WM, Gladstone H. Vascular foramina and arterial blood supply of the distal end of the femur. J Bone Joint Surg Am 1950;32(4):867–74.

[14] el Miedany YM, Wassif G, el Baddini M. Diffuse idiopathic skeletal hyperostosis (DISH): is it of vascular aetiology? Clin Exp Rheumatol 2000;18(2): 193–200.

[15] Failla JM. Hook of hamate vascularity: vulnerability to osteonecrosis and nonunion. J Hand Surg [Am] 1993; 18(6):1075–9.

[16] Fasol P, Munk P, Strickner M. Blood supply of the scaphoid bone of the hand. Acta Anat (Basel) 1978; 100(1):27–33.

[17] Lannigan FJ, O'Higgins P, McPhie P. The vascular supply of the lenticular and long processes of the incus. Clin Otolaryngol 1993;18(5):387–9.

[18] Longia GS, Ajmani ML, Saxena SK, et al. Study of diaphyseal nutrient foramina in human long bones. Acta Anat (Basel) 1980;107(4):399–406.

[19] Colles CM, Hickman J. The arterial blood supply of the navicular bone and its variations in navicular disease. Equine Vet J 1977;9(3):150–4.

[20] Jung A, Wurtz JP, Randrianarivo P. Les modifications circulatoires artérielles dans les nécroses aseptiques de la hanche et l'épiphysiolyse. Mémoires de l'Académie de Chirurgie 1965;91:489–506.

[21] Harty M. Symposium on surface replacement arthroplasty of the hip: anatomic consideration. Orthop Clin N Am 1982;13(4):667–79.

[22] Judet J, Judet R, Lagrange J, et al. A study of the vascularization of the femoral neck in the adult. J Bone Joint Surg Am 1955;37(4):663–80.

[23] Siebenrock KA, Ganz R. Osteochondroma of the femoral neck. Clin Orthop 2002;394:211–8.

[24] Siebenrock KA, Gautier E, Woo AK, et al. Surgical dislocation of the femoral head for joint debridement and accurate reduction of fractures of the acetabulum. J Orthop Trauma 2002;16(8):543–52.

[25] Beaule P. A soft tissue sparing approach for surface arthroplasty of the hip. Operat Tech Orthop 2004; 14(2):75–84.

[26] Campbell P, Mirra J, Amstutz HC. Viability of femoral heads treated with resurfacing arthroplasty. J Arthroplasty 2000;15(1):120–2.

[27] Grecula MJ, Grigoris P, Schmalzried TP, et al. Endoprostheses for osteonecrosis of the femoral head. A comparison of four models in young patients. Int Orthop 1995;19(3):137–43.

[28] Bradley GW, Freeman MA, Revell PA. Resurfacing arthroplasty. Femoral head viability. Clin Orthop 1987; 220:137–41.

[29] Freeman MA. Some anatomical and mechanical considerations relevant to the surface replacement of the femoral head. Clin Orthop 1978;134:19–24.

[30] Nelson EF, Matejcyzk MB, Greenwald AS, et al. Preliminary observations on the effects of surgical approach in surface replacement of the canine hip. Trans Orthop Res Soc 1980;5:177.

[31] Lange D, Whiteside L, Lesker P. Femoral head circulation: blood flow measurements in normal and arthritic canine femoral heads. Trans Orthop Res Soc 1979;4:14.

[32] Hedley A, Coster E, Amstutz H. The effects of vascular compromise on surface replacement of the hip—a canine model. Trans Orthop Res Soc 1980;5:176.

[33] Capello W, Wilson N, Wellman H. Bone imaging: a means of evaluating hip surface replacement arthroplasty. In: The hip: proceedings of the 8th Open Scientific Meeting of the Hip Society. St. Louis (MO): C.V. Mosby; 1980. p. 165–91.

[34] Whiteside LA, Lange DR, Capello WR, et al. The effects of surgical procedures on the blood supply to the femoral head. J Bone Joint Surg Am 1983;65(8):1127–33.

[35] Beaulé PE, Campbell P, Hoke R, et al. Femoral head vascularity and notching of the femoral neck during surface arthroplasty of the hip. Presented at the Orthopaedic Research Society meeting. Washington, DC, 2005.

[36] Siguier M, Judet T, Siguier T, et al. Preliminary results of partial surface replacement of the femoral head in osteonecrosis. J Arthroplasty 1999;14(1):45–51.

[37] Mont MA, Inhorn TA, Sponseller PD. The trapdoor procedure using autogenous cortical and cancellous bone grafts for osteonecrosis of the femoral head. J Bone Joint Surg Br 1998;80(1):56–62.

[38] Meyers M. The surgical treatment of osteonecrosis of the femoral hed with an osteochondral allograft. Acta Orthop Belg 1999;65(Suppl 1):66–7.

ELSEVIER
SAUNDERS

Orthop Clin N Am 36 (2005) 177 – 185

ORTHOPEDIC
CLINICS
OF NORTH AMERICA

Patient Selection and Surgical Technique for Surface Arthroplasty of the Hip

Paul E. Beaulé, MD, FRCSC[a,b,]*, John Antoniades, MD[b]

[a]*David Geffen School of Medicine at University of California Los Angeles, Los Angeles, CA, USA*
[b]*Joint Replacement Institute at Orthopaedic Hospital, 2400 S. Flower Street, Los Angeles, CA 90007, USA*

In recent years, there has been a resurgence in the interest of metal-on-metal surface arthroplasty of the hip [1] as an alternative to total hip replacement for the young and active adult [2]. Concomitantly, ceramic-on-ceramic bearings and new polyethylenes are being introduced as promising technology to improve the longevity of standard total hip replacements. Although these technologies are being embraced [3,4] by many, the 10-year survivorship of ceramic-on-ceramic total hips is relatively low at 79% to 85% [5,6] and the new polyethylenes have only 2-year data [7].

Similarly, the renewed interest in the clinically proven low wear of the metal-on-metal bearing [8,9] combined with the capacity of inserting a thin-wall cementless acetabular component [10] has fostered the reintroduction of surface arthroplasty of the hip. As in other forms of conservative hip surgery (ie, pelvic osteotomies [11] and surgical dislocation with femoral head-neck recontouring [12,13]), patient selection helps to minimize complications [14] and the need for early reoperation. Currently, there are two applications for hip resurfacing: hemiresurfacing in the early stages of osteonecrosis [15] and full-surface arthroplasty in the presence of advanced arthritis. In this article, current indications and surgical technique for surface arthroplasty for nonosteonecrotic hip pathology are reviewed.

Patient selection and current clinical results

There have been two recent publications on the short-term results of hybrid metal-on-metal surface arthroplasty that show 94% to 99.8% survivorship at 4 years [16,17]. In both series, patients returned to very high activity levels, with a mean patient age for both series of 48 years old. Amstutz and associates [16] identified several variables that put patients at risk for early failure: femoral head cysts, patient height, and previous hip surgery. In contrast, Daniel and associates [17] emphasized metallurgy and manufacturing of the metal-on-metal bearing as the main determinants for a well-functioning surface arthroplasty: hot isostatic pressing and solution annealing of the components were reported to be unfavorable to the wear properties [18]. Recent analysis and review of metal-on-metal bearings tested in hip simulators by Nevelos and associates [19], however, found no influence of the manufacturing process on the wear properties, with the main determinants for optimal wear performance being relatively low radial clearances and a high carbon content.

As with the introduction of cementless designs in total hip replacements [20], metal-on-metal bearings are not the only answer to the success of surface arthroplasty of the hip [21]. Beaulé et al [14] reviewed the short-term results of patients 40 years old and younger who underwent metal-on-metal surface arthroplasty and identified several independent factors that played a role in their premature failures. A Surface Arthroplasty Risk Index (SARI) was developed and based on a 6-point scoring system: femoral head cyst >1 cm = 2 points; weight <82 kg = 2 points; previous hip surgery = 1 point; and University of

---

* Corresponding author. David Geffen School of Medicine at University of California Los Angeles, Los Angeles, CA.

E-mail address: pbeaule@laoh.ucla.edu (P.E. Beaulé).

orthopedic.theclinics.com

California (UCLA) activity score >6 = 1 point. A SARI score >3 represented a 12-fold increase risk in early failure or adverse radiologic changes. In addition, when Amstutz and associates [16] reported on the overall experience in the first 400 hybrid metal-on-metal surface arthroplasties, patients with a SARI >3 had a survivorship of 89% at 4 years versus 97% with a score ≤3. The SARI also proved to be relevant in assessing the outcome of the all-cemented McMinn resurfacing implant (Corin, Ciren-cester, UK) at a mean follow-up of 8.7 years. Hips that had failed or had evidence of radiographic fail-ure on the femoral side had a significantly higher SARI score than the remaining hips (3.9 versus 1.9), with an overall survivorship at 7 years for the femo-ral and acetabular components of 93% and 80%, respectively [21].

In respect to the underlying diagnosis, initial analyses have not demonstrated any particular group at greater risk of early failure [16]. Structural ab-normalities present with certain diagnoses, however, might pose some difficulties in the positioning and fixation of the components. One such example is dysplasia in which the presence of an acetabular deficiency combined with the inability of inserting

screws through the acetabular component may make initial implant stability unpredictable. This deformity in combination with a significant leg-length discrep-ancy or valgus femoral neck could compromise the functional results after hip resurfacing, and in those situations, a stem-type total hip replacement may provide a superior functional outcome [22]. Surgeons must also consider the overall medical condition of the patient with respect to possible metal hypersen-tivity, which could cause persistent pain [23], and compromised renal function because metal ions gen-erated from the metal–metal bearing are excreted through the urine and the lack of clearance of these ions could lead to excessive levels in the blood [9,24].

Finally, as discussed earlier and due to the nega-tive effects of the development of a femoral head cyst on femoral fixation, intervention before the formation of a cyst within the femoral head should be con-sidered for surface arthroplasty of the hip (Fig. 1). This view is obviously contrary to the conventional wisdom of delaying a prosthetic solution for as long as possible; however, the advantages of a pain-free range of motion and maintaining normal activities without the need for anti-inflammatory medication

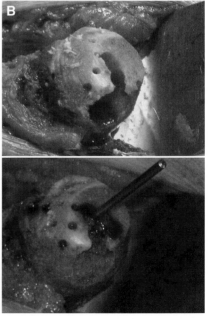

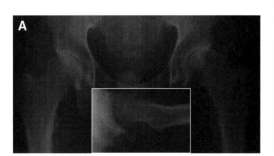

Fig. 1. (*A*) Forty-five-year-old man with an arthritic hip associated with a large femoral head cyst seen on anteroposterior radiograph and cross-table lateral radiograph (*inset*). (*B*) Intraoperative photographs after femoral head preparation showing the size of the cyst pre- (*upper panel*) and postgrafting (*lower panel*) with acetabular and femoral head reamings.

achieved with hip resurfacing cannot be ignored. This practice, combined with the known benefits of physical activity on one's overall health [25], may change how we perceive early prosthetic intervention with a conservative implant versus the inevitable decline associated with hip arthritis and side effects associated with chronic anti-inflammatory medication.

Surgical technique

Currently, the posterior approach is the most commonly used for hip resurfacing as presented by several authors within this issue of the *Orthopedic Clinics of North America*. As discussed by Nork and associates elsewhere in this issue, however, the choice of a surgical approach for hip resurfacing must factor in different anatomic considerations than when performing a standard total hip replacement. With preservation of the femoral head and neck, issues such as vascularity and adequate visualization with minimal trauma to tissues and nerves must be considered [10] (see Nork et al, this issue). For example, the choice of a surgical approach compromising femoral head blood supply [10,26] (see Nork et al, this issue) and causing osteonecrosis could lead to femoral loosening [27] or femoral neck fracture [28] if the lesion is sufficiently large. In addition, because of its conservative nature and goal to closely reproduce the normal anatomy of the proximal femur, positioning of the implants in hip resurfacing may have a greater impact on implant survivorship and patient function than with standard hip replacement.

In the 1982 *Orthopedic Clinics of North America* issue on surface arthroplasty, Hedley [26] emphasized the importance of maintaining femoral head vascularity when considering intervention in early stages of arthritis, whereas in the more advanced stages, an intramedullary source would be sufficient [29]. The discussion at that time was not so much on what surgical approach to use because most surgeons were using a pure anterior [30] or extracapsular trochanteric osteotomy [31], but whether one could safely dislocate the native hip joint without causing osteonecrosis. Subsequent retrieval analysis articles of failed surface arthroplasty failed to identify any major osteonecrotic segments [32–34]; however, the massive granulomatous reaction from the polyethylene wear debris combined with bone resorption secondary to implant micromotion did not leave much of the bone intact at the implant interface. More important, most surgeons at that time were performing hip resurfacing through approaches that left the ob-

turator externus tendon intact, protecting the branch of the medial circumflex artery [35]. In addition, there is recent evidence that the blood supply pattern in advanced arthritis is not significantly different than in the nonarthritic state [36]. Recent work on arthritic femoral heads presented at the annual Orthopaedic Research Society meeting in Washington, DC demonstrated using laser doppler flowmetry that damage to the extraosseous blood supply to the femoral head (retinacular vessels) can cause a significant decrease (greater than 50%) in blood flow [36]. Further follow-up and research is required before the role of femoral head vascularity on the clinical outcome of hip resurfacing can be fully assessed; however, the choice of a surgical approach that minimizes the risk of damaging the blood supply to the femoral head needs to be strongly considered. This choice may become even more crucial as surgeons consider cementless fixation on the femoral side and earlier intervention in the arthritic process to avoid the development of femoral head cysts.

In sharp contrast to stem-type total hip replacements, femoral component positioning in the coronal and the sagittal/axial planes has a narrower margin of error and is dependent on the surgical technique [37] and influenced by the underlying pathology/deformity that led to the degenerative changes. In the coronal plane, varus placement should be avoided, with a relative valgus of 5° to 10° degrees minimizing the tensile stresses at the superior bone–prosthesis junction [29,37]. For example, placement of the femoral component at 130° compared with 140° would increase the tensile stresses by 31%. In the sagittal/axial plane, restoring or maintaining head-neck offset is different than with a stem-type total hip replacement. Although impingement after total hip replacement has long been recognized to limit range of motion [38] and, in extreme cases, lead to hip instability [39], the risk after surface arthroplasty may be greater because the femoral head-neck unit is preserved. This is particularly true in hips in which the arthritis was secondary to femoro acetabular impingement [40]. This common cause of hip arthritis is felt to be secondary to a lack of femoral head-neck offset in the anterolateral area of the femoral head-neck junction [41–43]. If this pathology is left unrecognized after surface arthroplasty of the hip, patients could still experience impingement between the rim of the acetabulum or with the acetabular component itself [44] or have a restricted range of motion. Thus, at the time of resurfacing arthroplasty, removal of prominent anterior neck osteophytes or anterior translation of the femoral component should be considered to avoid this phenomenon [10].

To illustrate some of these different technical points, a series of four case illustrations is presented. The authors do not discuss the detailed surgical technique, which has been described elsewhere [1,10]. The implant used by the senior author (P.E.B.) is the Conserve Plus design (Wright Medical Technology, Memphis, Tennessee) manufactured from high carbon cast cobalt-chromium-molybdenum conforming to ASTM F75 standards. It is available in sizes from 36 to 54 mm in 2-mm increments. Two shell sizes are available in terms of wall thickness: 3.5 mm (thin shell) and 5.0 mm (thick shell). The femoral component has a short stem to ensure accurate alignment, with a uniform cement mantle around the resurfaced femoral head. To provide some cement mantle for the short stem, the authors recommend over-reaming by 2 mm with the stem reamer. No data are yet available on how cementing the short stem may improve long-term survivorship, but the authors have not seen any

negative effects [45]. Finally, it is unclear what the optimal cement mantle is on the femoral side because recommendations and designs vary between manufacturers. For example, the Conserve Plus and the DuROM (Zimmer, Warsaw, Indiana) tend to have a thicker mantle than the Birmingham Hip Resurfacing (Smith Nephew, Memphis, Tennessee) and the Cormet 2000 (Corin, Cirencester, UK) designs. In the latter two designs, this thinner mantle results in deeper penetration of the cement into the femoral head.

In terms of surgical approach, the senior author (P.E.B.) adopted the digastric approach with trochanteric slide osteotomy [10], which defers slightly from Ganz et al's description [12] in terms of the exposure of the acetabulum during its preparation: the leg is kept in slight flexion with the knee in extension. Because this approach is done through tissue that allows effective apposition during the healing phase and the only fascia that is cut and repaired in tension

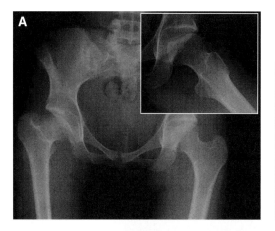
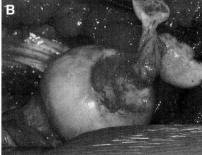
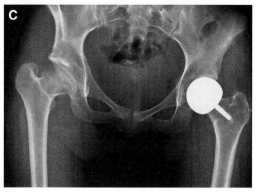

Fig. 2. (*A*) Anteroposterior radiograph and frog lateral radiograph (*inset*) showing the large osteochonral defect of the weight-bearing area of the femoral head. (*B*) Intraoperative photograph showing the femoral head before preparation. (*C*) Anteroposterior radiograph 18 months posthemiresurfacing arthroplasty.

is that between the gluteus maximus and the tensor fasciae lata, it causes no damage intentional or otherwise, to muscles. Thus, not only is this approach less invasive from an implant/bone resection standpoint but it also minimizes soft tissue trauma and facilitates a return to normal function. The trochanteric fragment is usually fixed with two to three 3.5-mm screws, with 50% weight bearing for 4 to 6 weeks, at which time physical therapy is initiated.

Case illustrations

Sequelae of Legg-Calvé-Perthes disease

A 20-year-old woman presented with a history of Legg-Calvé-Perthes disease involving both hips at the age of 9 years. She underwent a pelvic osteotomy on the right hip at the age of 12 years with no treatment on the left hip. She presented with a 1-year history of increasing left hip pain with no associated trauma. This pain was also associated with a clicking and catching in her hip. On physical examination, she had an antalgic gait with some restriction in range of motion, with a positive impingement test. Plain radiographs revealed a large osteochondral defect with no evidence of arthritis (Fig. 2A). Femoral head allograft reconstruction and hemiresurfacing arthroplasty were discussed. The patient elected to undergo the hemiresurfacing arthroplasty. At the time of surgical intervention, there was a large femoral defect with a

loose osteochondral fragment (Fig. 2B). Using suture anchors, the labrum was repaired to re-establish the fluid seal in the hip joint. A super-finished Conserve Plus femoral component was cemented in placed after appropriate sizing (Fig. 2C). The screws were removed at 1 year. At 18 months' follow-up, the patient is functioning well with pain only after long periods of standing or use of high heels.

This case illustrates the use of the Conserve Plus super-finished femoral component as a hemiresurfacing component that can later be converted to full-surface arthroplasty, leaving the femoral component in situ. In terms of surgical technique, alignment of the femoral component within the anatomic neck axis was done to minimize joint reaction forces on the acetabular cartilage, thus a valgus orientation was purposely avoided [37].

Protrusio acetabuli

A 17-year-old boy presented with severe pain in the left hip for 1 year, requiring the use of crutches for ambulation. His range of motion was restricted, with only 70° of flexion and 15° of rotational arc. His right hip was asymptomatic (Fig. 3A). The acetabulum was reconstructed with a modular cementless shell, and the femoral component was cemented. Allomatrix (Wright Medical Technology) with reamings of the femoral head were used to graft the medial wall deficiency. At 1-year post surgery, the patient returned to his normal activities, with both hips being asymptomatic (Fig. 3B).

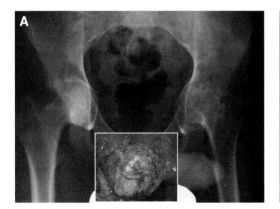 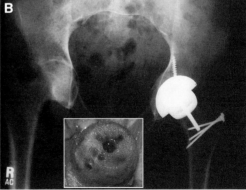

Fig. 3. (A) Anteroposterior radiograph showing the protrusio deformity and destruction of the left hip joint. Inset is an intraoperative picture of the femoral head. (B) One-year postoperative anteroposterior radiograph showing a well-fixed hybrid metal-on-polyethylene hip resurfacing arthroplasty. Inset photograph shows the femoral head after preparation. The acetabulum was reconstructed with a modular cementless shell (58-mm outside diameter; Trabecular Metal Cup, Zimmer, Warsaw, IN) and a highly cross-linked polyethylene (40-mm inner diameter; Longevity, Zimmer).

To restore the hip center and correct the pincer type of femoroacetabular impingement [40], grafting and supplementary screw fixation of the acetabulum was necessary. In this situation, the use of a modular acetabular component was used, permitting the use of two possible femoral component sizes: 36 mm and 40 mm. The current wear properties and early clinical results of the new highly cross-linked polyethylenes [7,46] make them a reasonable alternative to the metal-on-metal bearing in cases where the acetabulum has sufficient capacity for the acetabular component. On the femoral side, because the 40-mm component was the largest that could be used and to prevent notching of the femoral neck and excessive thinning of the head-neck junction, the authors stopped the reaming down at 42 mm and cemented a 40-mm femoral component. With the Conserve Plus system and despite under reaming, the femoral component can be fully seated but with a thinner cement mantle.

Insufficient head-neck offset

A 40-year-old man presented with a 5-year history of right hip pain that had worsened in the last 8 months. There was no history of childhood hip disorders or significant traumatic events. The patient had been a professional skateboarder and wanted to return to that sport and to snowboarding. His other hip was asymptomatic. On preoperative radiographs, the hip had a classic pistol grip appearance, with an offset ratio on the cross-table lateral of 0.10 (Fig. 4A). This ratio is calculated by dividing the anterior offset by the head diameter [42]. The patient underwent metal-on-metal resurfacing arthroplasty and at 2 years post surgery is back to professional skateboarding and winter sports. On the postoperative cross-table lateral, the offset ratio was improved to 0.22 (Fig. 4B).

Posttraumatic

A 32-year-old man developed avascular necrosis and posttraumatic arthritis after open reduction and internal fixation for an acetabular fracture sustained in a motor vehicle accident 4 years ago. The patient now had constant pain in his hip, significantly restricting his ambulation that was further limited by a leg-length discrepancy of 2 cm and partial peroneal nerve palsy. Radiographs including Judet obliques revealed retained internal fixation on both columns with loss of acetabular bone stock (Fig. 5A, B). After appropriate consultation and discussion of other options such as hip arthrodesis [47], the patient elected to undergo a metal-on-metal surface arthroplasty of the hip. The patient underwent removal of the hardware through an ilioinguinal approach and insertion of the metal–metal surface arthoplasty through the trochanteric slide osteotomy. The leg-length correction was achieved by restoring the hip center with a porous, beaded acetabular component (Conserve Plus), providing a secure initial press-fit without the need for adjunct fixation.

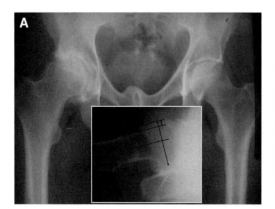
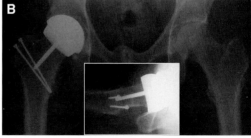

Fig. 4. (*A*) Anteroposterior radiograph showing aspherical femoral head with advanced arthritic changes. Inset demonstrates offset ratio measurement on the cross-table lateral radiograph. (*B*) Postoperative anteroposterior radiograph at 2 years post metal-on-metal hip resurfacing. Inset shows appropriate offset restoration on the cross-table lateral radiograph.

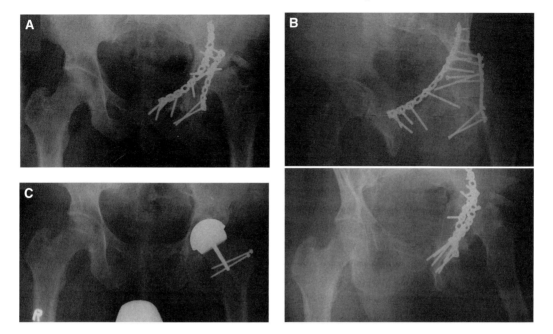

Fig. 5. (*A*) Anteroposterior radiogaph demonstrating the femoral head deformity and leg-length discrepancy. (*B*) The Judet 45° obliques demonstrate that the roof of the acetabulum is deficient but the anterior and posterior columns are relatively intact. (*C*) Anteroposterior radiograph post hybrid resurfacing arthroplasty.

At 2 years, the patient is doing well with minimal pain. Radiographs reveal a correction of the initial leg-length discrepancy and no evidence of component loosening (Fig. 5C).

Summary

The last symposium that was published on surface arthroplasty of the hip [48] concluded that surface arthroplasty should not be considered a standard arthroplasty, should be performed only by surgeons with considerable experience in hip reconstruction, and should be considered in the stage of evaluation. These conclusions are still true today. For surface arthroplasty of the hip to be considered a viable alternative to total hip replacement, certain goals must be met: achieve survivorship superior to 90% at 5 to 10 years, prove itself as a reproducible technique, and confirm its ease of conversion to total hip replacement. Finally, preserving femoral head vascularity by careful surgical technique needs to be considered to optimize the long-term outcome and permit intervention earlier in the arthritic process.

References

[1] Beaule PE, Amstutz HC. Surface arthroplasty of the hip revisited: current indications and surgical technique. In: Sinha RJ, editor. Hip replacement: current trends and controversies. New York: Marcel Dekker; 2002. p. 261–97.

[2] Sochart DH. Relationship of acetabular wear to osteolysis and loosening in total hip arthroplasty. Clin Orthop 1999;363:135–50.

[3] D'Antonio JA, Capello WN, Manley M, et al. New experience with alumina-on-alumina ceramic bearings for total hip arthroplasty. J Arthroplasty 2002;17(4): 390–7.

[4] Garino JP. Modern ceramic-on-ceramic total hip systems in the United States. Clin Orthop 2000;379: 41–7.

[5] Hamadouche M, Boutin P, Daussange J, et al. Alumina-on-alumina total hip arthroplasty: a minimum 18.5-year follow-up study. J Bone Joint Surg [Am] 2002;84(1):69–77.

[6] Bizot P, Banallec L, Sedel L, et al. Alumina-on-alumina total hip prostheses in patients 40 years of age or younger. Clin Orthop 2000;379:68–76.

[7] Heisel C, Silva M, dela Rosa M, et al. Short-term in vivo wear of cross-linked polyethylenes. J Bone Joint Surg [Am] 2004;86(4):748–51.

[8] Sieber H-P, Rieker CB, Kottig P. Analysis of 118 second-generation metal-on-metal retrieved hip implants. J Bone Joint Surg [Br] 1999;81(1):46–50.

[9] Brodner W, Bitzan P, Meisinger V, et al. Serum cobalt levels after metal-on-metal total hip arthroplasty. J Bone Joint Surg [Am] 2003;85(11):2168–73.

[10] Beaulé PE. A soft tissue sparing approach to surface arthroplasty of the hip. Oper Tech Ortho 2004;14(4):16–8.

[11] Trousdale RT, Ekkernkamp A, Ganz R, et al. Periacetabular and intertrochanteric osteotomy for the treatment of osteoarthrosis in dysplastic hips. J Bone Joint Surg [Am] 1995;77(1):73–85.

[12] Ganz R, Gill TJ, Gautier E, et al. Surgical dislocation of the adult hip. A new technique with full access to the femoral head and acetabulum without the risk of avascular necrosis. J Bone Joint Surg [Br] 2001;83(8):1119–24.

[13] Beck M, Leunig M, Parvizi J, et al. Anterior femoroacetabular impingement. Part II. Midterm results of surgical treatment. Clin Orthop 2004;418:67–73.

[14] Beaulé PE, Dorey FJ, LeDuff MJ, et al. Risk factors affecting outcome of metal on metal surface arthroplasty of the hip. Clin Orthop 2004;418:87–93.

[15] Beaulé PE, Amstutz HC. Treatment of Ficat stage III and IV osteonecrosis of the hip. J Am Acad Orthop Surg 2004;12(2):96–105.

[16] Amstutz HC, Beaulé PE, Dorey FJ, et al. Metal-on-metal hybrid surface arthroplasty: two to six year follow-up. J Bone Joint Surg [Am] 2004;86(1):28–39.

[17] Daniel J, Pynsent PB, McMinn DJW. Metal-on-metal resurfacing of the hip in patients under the age of 55 years with osteoarthritis. J Bone Joint Surg [Br] 2004;86(2):177–84.

[18] McMinn DJW. Development of metal/metal hip resurfacing. Hip Int 2003;13(1 Suppl 2):S41–53.

[19] Nevelos J, Shelton JC, Fisher J. Metallurgical considerations in the wear of metal-on-metal hip bearings. Hip Int 2004;14(1):1–10.

[20] Jones LC, Hungerford DS. Cement disease. Clin Orthop 1987;225:192–206.

[21] Beaulé PE, LeDuff M, Campbell P, et al. Metal-on-metal surface arthroplasty with a cemented femoral component: a 7–10 year followup study. J Arthroplasty 2004;19(8 Suppl 3):17–22.

[22] Silva M, Lee KH, Heisel C., et al. The biomechanical results of total hip resurfacing arthroplasty. J Bone Joint Surg [Am] 2004;86(1):40–1.

[23] Willert H-G, Buchhorn GH, Fayyazi A, et al. Metal-on-metal bearings and hypersensitivity in patients with artifical hip joints. A clinical and histomorphological study. J Bone Joint Surg [Am] 2005;87(1):28–36.

[24] Jacobs J, Skipor A, Doorn P, et al. Cobalt and chromium concentrations in patients with metal on metal total hip replacements. Clin Orthop 1996;329S:S256–63.

[25] Paffenbarger RS, Hyde RT, Wing AL, et al. Physical activity, all-cause mortality, and longevity of college alumni. N Engl J Med 1986;314(10):605–13.

[26] Hedley AK. Technical considerations with surface replacement. Orthop Clin N [Am] 1982;13(4):747–60.

[27] Bell RS, Schatzker J, Fornasier VL, et al. A study of implant failure in the Wagner resurfacing arthroplasty. J Bone Joint Surg [Am] 1985;67:1165–75.

[28] Amstutz HC, Le Duff MJ, Campbell PA. Fracture of the neck of the femur after surface arthroplasty of the hip. J Bone Joint Surg [Am] 2004;86(9):1874–7.

[29] Freeman MAR. Some anatomical and mechanical considerations relevant to the surface replacement of the femoral head. Clin Orthop 1978;134:19–24.

[30] Wagner H. Surface replacement arthroplasty of the hip. Clin Orthop 1978;134:102–30.

[31] Amstutz HC, Graff-Radford A, Mai L, et al. Surface replacement of the hip with the THARIES system. J Bone Joint Surg [Am] 1981;63(7):1069–77.

[32] Howie DW, Cornish BL, Vernon-Roberts B. The viability of the femoral head after resurfacing hip arthroplasty in humans. Clin Orthop 1993;291:171–84.

[33] Campbell PA, Mirra J, Amstutz HC. Viability of femoral head treated with resurfacing arthroplasty. J Arthroplasty 2000;15(1):120–2.

[34] Freeman MA, Bradley GW. ICLH surface replacement of the hip. An analysis of the first 10 years. J Bone Joint Surg [Br] 1983;65(4):405–11.

[35] Gautier E, Ganz K, Krugel N, et al. Anatomy of the medial circumflex artery and its surgical implications. J Bone Joint Surg [Br] 2000;82(5):679–83.

[36] Beaule PE, Campbell PA, Hoke R. Femoral head vascularity and notching of the femoral neck during surface arthroplasty of the hip. Washington, DC: Orthopaedic Research Society; 2005.

[37] Beaule PE, Lee J, LeDuff M, et al. Orientation of femoral component in surface arthroplasty of the hip: a biomechanical and clinical analysis. J Bone Joint Surg [Am] 2004;86(9):2015–21.

[38] Amstutz HC, Markolf KL. Design features in total hip replacement. In: Harris WH, editor. Proceedings of the Hip Society. St. Louis (MO): The Hip Society; 1974. p. 111–24.

[39] Bartz RL, Noble PC, Kadakia NR, et al. The effect of femoral component head size on posterior dislocation of the artificial hip joint. J Bone Joint Surg [Am] 2000;82(9):1300–7.

[40] Ganz R, Parvizi J, Leunig M, et al. Femoroacetabular Impingement: a cause for osteoarthritis of the hip. Clin Orthop 2003;417:112–20.

[41] Ito K, Minka-II MA, Leunig S, et al. Femoroacetabular impingement and the cam-effect. J Bone Joint Surg [Br] 2001;83(2):171–6.

[42] Eijer H, Leunig M, Mahomed N, et al. Cross-table lateral radiographs for screening of anterior femoral head-neck offset in patients with femoro-acetabular impingement. Hip Int 2001;11(1):37–41.

[43] Beaulé PE, Zaragoza EJ, Copelan N. 3-Dimensional computer tomography in the assessment of femoroacetabular impingement. San Francisco (CA): Orthopaedic Research Society; 2004.

[44] Wiadrowski TP, McGee M, Cornish BL, et al. Periph-

eral wear of Wagner resurfacing hip arthroplasty acetabular components. J Arthroplasty 1991;6(2):103–7.

[45] Amstutz HC, Beaulé PE, LeDuff MJ. Hybrid metal-on-metal surface arthroplasty of the hip. Oper Tech Ortho 2001;11(4):253–62.

[46] Digas G, Karrholm J, Thanner J, et al. Highly cross-linked polyethylene in total hip arthroplasty: randomized evaluation of penetration rate in cemented and uncemented sockets using radiostereometric analysis. Clin Orthop 2004;429:6–16.

[47] Beaule PE, Matta JM, Mast JW. Hip arthrodesis: current indications and techniques. J Am Acad Orthop Surg 2002;10:249–58.

[48] Steinberg ME. Summary and conclusions: Symposium on Surface Replacement Arthroplasty of the Hip. Orthop Clin N [Am] 1982;13(4):895–902.

ELSEVIER
SAUNDERS

Orthop Clin N Am 36 (2005) 187–193

ORTHOPEDIC
CLINICS
OF NORTH AMERICA

Complications Associated with Hip Resurfacing Arthroplasty

A.J. Shimmin, MBBS, FRACS, Dip Anat*, J. Bare, MBBS, FRACS,
D.L. Back, FRCS(Edin)(Orth)

The Melbourne Orthopaedic Group, 33 The Avenue Windsor, 3181 Melbourne, Australia

Hip resurfacing arthroplasty is an old orthopedic concept that has undergone a resurgence of interest in the past decade [1–8]. Previous problems associated with thin polyethylene acetabular components, reproducible quality of manufacturing of metal-on-metal implants, and component fixation issues appear to have been resolved and a more reliable prosthesis developed [4,8,9].

The proposed advantages of hip resurfacing over conventional total hip arthroplasty are bone conservation, reproduction of anatomic hip biomechanics, greater implant stability, and assumed easier revision procedures.

There are no long-term results available on the new-generation hip resurfacing arthroplasties. Studies of the Conserve Plus (Wright Medical Technology, Arlington, Tennessee), the McMinn and Cormet (Corin Medical, Cirencester, UK), and the Birmingham Hip Resurfacing (Midland Medical Technologies, Birmingham, UK) have a mean of 3 years' follow-up demonstrating survivorship of >97% [1,2, 10]. These studies demonstrate significantly better survivorship than previous generations of hip resurfacing prostheses (eg, Wagner, Imperial College London Hospital (ICLH), THARIES, Furaya) [1,6,7]. The most popular prosthesis currently in use is the Birmingham Hip Resurfacing.

Over the last decade, there has been a rapid increase in the number of procedures being performed,

and previously recognized complications have begun to recur; for example, femoral neck fracture [1,6,7]. Our understanding of these problems is continuously evolving, allowing us to better inform patients of the risks and allow further development of the technology to try to overcome them [11].

The ideal candidate for a hip resurfacing procedure is currently believed to be a young (<60 years) active man with normal proximal femoral bone geometry and bone quality who would be expected to outlive any current conventional prosthesis. Preoperative diagnoses can be varied and include osteoarthritis, osteonecrosis, and degenerative conditions secondary to developmental hip dysplasia, slipped capital femoral epiphysis, and Legg-Calvé-Perthes disease.

Contraindications for a resurfacing procedure are still being defined. Currently, absolute contraindications include elderly people with osteoporotic proximal femoral bone, known metal hypersensitivity, and impaired renal function. Relative contraindications include inflammatory arthropathies, severe acetabular dysplasia, grossly abnormal proximal femoral geometry (as may be encountered with some severe cases of Legg-Calvé-Perthes and slipped capital femoral epiphysis), large areas of avascular necrosis, and large geode formation (Fig. 1).

Problems that have been encountered can be divided into two main groups: (1) those associated with any type of hip arthroplasty; for example, dislocation, thromboembolic disease, heterotopic ossification, nerve palsies, and vascular damage; and (2) those that are more specifically related to the hip resurfacing procedure and the focus of this article; namely, femoral neck fractures, avascular necrosis, raised

* Corresponding author.
E-mail address: ashimmin@optusnet.com.au
(A.J. Shimmin).

0030-5898/05/$ – see front matter © 2005 Elsevier Inc. All rights reserved.
doi:10.1016/j.ocl.2005.01.002

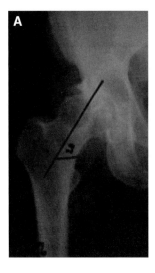
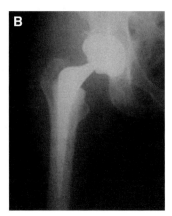

Fig. 1. (A) A case deemed unsuitable for hip resurfacing due to a large femoral head cyst that would compromise femoral component fixation and mechanics. (B) Postoperative radiograph.

metal ion levels, and sound initial and durable long-term fixation of an all-metal monoblock cobalt/chrome acetabular component.

Femoral neck fracture

Retention of the femoral neck exposes the patient to the risk of femoral neck fracture in the immediate postoperative period and in the future as per the general aging population.

A recently conducted multisurgeon national audit of the first 3429 Birmingham Hip Resurfacings, performed over a 4-year period, demonstrated a femoral neck fracture rate of 1.46% (50 cases). The fate of all inserted prostheses was known. Mean time to fracture was 15.4 weeks (range 0–56 weeks) [12]. Important patient, surgical, and postoperative factors with regard to the risk of fracture were identified from this review.

Patient factors

Patient factors included sex and proximal femoral bone quality. The national fracture rate was 0.98% for men and 1.91% for women undergoing hip resurfacing. This difference was statistically significant (χ^2 test: $P < 0.001$); that is, women were twice as likely to fracture as men. No conclusions could be drawn with regard to the optimum age range for a hip resurfacing from this audit. It may be postulated, however, that the decrease in bone density in postmenopausal women may have been a factor [12].

Surgical factors

Surgical factors associated with an increased risk of femoral neck fracture included notching of the superior femoral neck cortex (Fig. 2) combined with varus placement of the femoral component relative to the anatomic femoral neck shaft angle. In this series, 26 of 50 cases demonstrated notching of the femoral neck on the postoperative radiograph and 42 of 50 cases had a varus-placed femoral prosthesis [12,13].

When consenting the patient for a hip resurfacing procedure, it is advisable to also consent for a total hip arthroplasty. If problems are encountered with alignment, notching, or large geode formation, then conversion to a conventional hip arthroplasty is an option.

This evidence is consistent with known biomechanical considerations as proposed by Freeman [13] and knowledge gained from a recent retrospective biomechanical and clinical analysis [14] of 94 hips with a mean follow-up of 4.2 years. The resultant force vectors borne by the femoral head during walking encounter the femoral head at an angle of approximately 20° to the vertical in the frontal plane. The medial trabecular system lies in this axis. It has been shown that the strongest bone in compression is that of the medial trabecular system, whereas the bone in the head medial to this system is weak.

Hence, in the varus position, (1) tensile stresses appear in the bone of the lateral surface of the neck as it enters the prosthesis, (2) the medial compressive stresses rise considerably, and (3) sheer stresses develop at the mouth of the prosthesis [11].

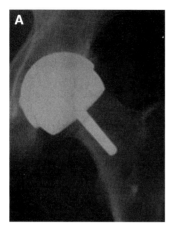 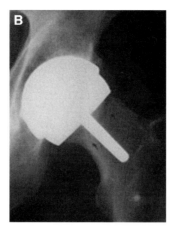 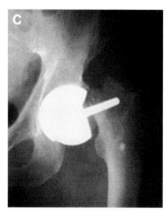

Fig. 2. (*A*) Postoperative radiograph of a femoral head prepared with a notch in the superior neck that may have contributed to the propagation of a fracture as seen evolving 6 weeks post surgery (*B*) and 10 weeks post surgery (*C*).

Postoperative factors

All patients in this national audit [12] were instructed to mobilize fully weight bearing postoperatively. Because the femoral neck undergoes a considerable surgical insult from intramedullary instrumentation, cylindrical reaming, and chamfer cutting, it may be reasonable to surmise that this treatment results in a "stressed" femur. A period of protected weight bearing postoperatively may reduce any tendency to fracture, particularly if notching of the femoral neck has occurred.

Avascular necrosis of the femoral head

In theory, preparation of the femoral head could cause avascular necrosis, which could ultimately lead to failure of the prosthesis due to loosening or periprosthetic fracture. Freeman [13] believed that the arthritic hip undergoes changes in the vascular supply of the femoral head, with the blood supply being predominantly intraosseous in arthritic hips rather than subsynovial vessels [11]. Current studies report a low incidence of avascular necrosis as a cause of implant failure at a mean of 3 years [1–3]. Studies on isolated primary hemiresurfacing of the femoral head report an absence of avascular necrosis on retrieval specimens [15]. These series appear to support Freeman's [13] theories.

The choice of surgical approach is theoretically an issue in the development of avascular necrosis. Traditionally, the posterior approach has been the most commonly used. This approach sacrifices the ascending branch of the medial femoral circumflex artery, which is an important contributor to the subsynovial supply of the normal femoral head. More recently, some surgeons have adopted the direct lateral or the surgical dislocation approach popularized by Ganz et al [16,17].

Other possible reasons for the small incidence of avascular necrosis with resurfacing procedures may reflect that it is the neck rather than the head that is being resurfaced. Considering that the technique involves resecting a portion of the zenith of the head and pressurizing cement for several millimeters into the prepared surface, it may be that there is not much remaining of the bone proximal to the fused epiphyseal plate. This allows us to conclude that it is the intraosseous femoral neck blood supply that is of paramount importance.

Metal ion levels

Hip resurfacing has the requirement to produce a thin acetabular shell of between 3 and 5 mm. This measurement limits the material of choice to metal-on-metal bearings.

Metal-on-metal bearings have been used in orthopedic surgery for the hip for the past 40 years and there have been no conclusive studies to suggest that they cause any adverse long-term effects (ie, carcinogenesis) [18–22]. It is known that metal-on-metal bearings produce higher serum cobalt and chromium levels than conventional metal-on-polyethylene bearings. Numerous articles have shown elevation of metal ion levels in metal-on-metal articulations compared with other articulations [23–26]; however, it is difficult to compare series because they measure different combinations of parameters (serum, blood, erythrocyte, and urine) using different measurement techniques. These different techniques have a wide range of sensitivities and baseline measurements. In addition, the significance of these elevated levels is not known.

Recent prospective studies of the Birmingham Hip Resurfacing have shown that serum cobalt levels rise to a peak at 6 months post procedure and are still declining at 3 years. The chromium levels peak at 9 months and then begin to decline. In these patients, no clinical issues appear to relate to the serum ion elevation in the short-term [27]; however, sporadic cases of hypersensitivity are being seen. Whether this is a true hypersensitivity response or a capsular response to a toxic local concentration of metal ion is unclear [28,29].

Hallab's [30–33] metal sensitivity work suggests that (1) the incidence of dermatologic sensitivities to metals in arthroplasty patients is higher than in the general population; (2) the risk of sensitivity to orthopedic implants is minimal and it is unclear whether metal sensitivity contributes to implant failure; and (3) preoperative dermatologic screening for metal hypersensitivity (delayed-type) is unreliable for predicting the response to a metallic prosthesis.

Currently, there is no reliable hematologic preoperative test to predict hypersensitivity, although work is being done on the development of lymphocyte reactivity tests to the alloy used in these implants [30–33].

The new generation of hip resurfacings are all formed from cobalt/chrome alloys. Different implants vary subtly in design and manufacturing processes. Whether implant manufacturing issues (ie, cast versus wrought cobalt/chromium, heat treating versus no heat treating, or variations in radial clearance) will influence the incidence of hypersensitivity/toxicity responses will become apparent with more detailed long-term follow-up of these implants [34].

The issues surrounding metal ion levels can be removed as a concern when ceramic bearings can be manufactured in the required dimensions.

Acetabular component fixation

In the absence of wear particles generating osteolysis, femoral component failure and loosening may result from fracture or avascular necrosis. Issues surrounding acetabular component aseptic loosening are somewhat different.

Initial reports on a pilot study by McMinn et al [2] that compared different forms of fixation in hip resurfacing arthroplasty found that hydroxyapatite-coated acetabular components gave the best clinical and radiographic outcomes. More recent reports on the results of the McMinn hybrid resurfacing and the Birmingham Hip Resurfacing arthroplasty have a mean follow-up of 3.3 years (range, 1.1–8.2 years) [3]. There are 446 hips in this series, and so far, there have been no reported acetabular-related failures. Amstutz et al [1] also recently published a series of 400 Conserve Plus hips. This group has an average follow-up of 3.5 years (range, 2.2–6.2 years). Only

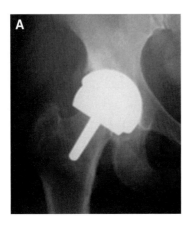 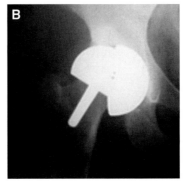

Fig. 3. (*A*) Radiograph taken 12 months post implantation. The patient was fully functional and very happy. (*B*) Radiograph taken 18 months post implantation when the patient presented with acute onset of groin pain after rising from a chair.

one hip (0.3%) has been revised for early failure of the acetabular component; however, a 32% rate of radiolucency (26% in one zone, 6% in two zones) was also reported. The clinical significance of these findings remains to be seen.

Good long-term success has been reported with cementless acetabular fixation in total hip arthroplasty [35–37]. Aseptic failures of these cups have largely been attributed to osteolysis from high volumetric polyethylene wear debris, a problem theoretically reduced by removing polyethylene from resurfacing arthroplasty [5]. A number of differences exist between the acetabular component of a total hip arthroplasty and that of a resurfacing arthroplasty that could lead to poorer results in the resurfacing group:

1. All modern hip resurfacing arthroplasties use a solid cobalt/chromium cup of between 3 and 5 mm thickness. Theoretically, because titanium is more biocompatible and has a modulus of elasticity closer to bone than cobalt/chromium, it should allow greater osseointegration. Therefore, most cementless total hip replacement systems use titanium as the ingrowth surface for the acetabular component [38–42]. Whether concern about biologic fixation of cementless cobalt/chromium cups is a theoretic rather than practical problem will evolve with ongoing long-term clinical review of large series (Fig. 3).
2. The inability to place screws behind the bearing surface increases the requirement to attain a secure initial press-fit fixation. To limit this potential problem, some resurfacing acetabular components provide supplementary fixation in the form of fins, peripheral expansion, or cups with peripheral screw holes such as the Birmingham dysplasia cup.

Other complications

Due to the larger-sized femoral component and because of restoring anatomic hip biomechanics, the rate of dislocation of a hip resurfacing prosthesis appears to be significantly less than that of a conventional total hip arthroplasty [43]. Published dislocation rates are 0.75% at a mean of 3 years' follow-up. In an initial series of 231 cases, there were no dislocations [1,3,44].

The reported rates of deep venous thrombosis, pulmonary embolus, heterotopic bone, and intraoperative nerve and vessel injury [44] are comparable with traditional arthroplasty techniques.

Summary

Hip resurfacing surgery is an evolving field in orthopedics. The complications discussed can be summarized as having a combination of causes. Surgical factors are undoubtedly important and involve preoperative and intraoperative decision making and surgical technique. Other, less controllable complications are due to biologic and material factors.

Periprosthetic fracture of the femoral neck is the most common complication. Its cause is multifactorial, including patient selection, surgical technique, and postoperative management. Avascular necrosis has occurred but is less frequent than might be expected when using the traditional posterior approach for this procedure. It is thought that the osteoarthritic hip develops a more intraosseous blood supply throughout the course of this disease, placing it at lower risk of developing avascular necrosis subsequent to any resurfacing procedure.

Elevated serum and blood metal ion levels and local tissue toxicity or hypersensitivity are other potential problems of this procedure, which currently still requires the use of a metal-on-metal articulation. Despite a long history of the use of metal-on-metal articulations with no proven adverse clinical consequences, concerns are still expressed with regard to the long-term outcome of elevated serum metal ion levels. There also are some sporadic cases of local hypersensitivity/toxicity. Preoperative lymphocyte reactivity tests may help to predict susceptible individuals in the future.

Aseptic loosening of the acetabular component may occur at later follow-up because of the rigidity of the implant and poorer bone ingrowth at the acetabular interface. Newer designs have titanium surface finishes to theoretically provide better osseous integration of the acetabular component.

Dislocation rates after resurfacing are predictably lower than for conventional 28-mm head total hip replacements due to the larger head size and more accurate restoration of hip biomechanics.

Currently, there are no survivorship figures to assess the long-term prognosis of this procedure, although initial results appear promising. Of the new generation of hip resurfacings, there have been only two short-term (3-year) reviews published, which have come from the designers of the two prostheses [1,3].

There is a need for independent prospective studies to be published in the orthopedic literature to allow better guidance on this procedure. More publications will allow better assessment of complication rates and the suitability of this prosthesis for long-term use.

References

[1] Amstutz HC, Beaule PE, Dorey FJ, et al. Metal-on-metal hybrid surface arthropasty: two to six year follow up study. J Bone Joint Surg [Am] 2004;86(1): 28–39.

[2] McMinn D, Treacy R, Lin K, et al. Metal on metal surface replacement of the hip. Experience of the McMinn prosthesis. Clin Orthop 1996;329S:S89–98.

[3] Daniel J, Pynsent PB, McMinn DJW. Metal on metal resurfacing of the hip in patients under the age of 55 years with osteoarthritis. J Bone Joint Surg [Br] 2004;86:177–84.

[4] Amstutz HC, Dorey FJ, O'Carroll PF. THARIES resurfacing arthroplasty. Clin Orthop 1986;213:92–113.

[5] Amstutz HC, Grigoris P, Dorey FJ. Evolution and future of surface replacement of the hip. J Orthop Sci 1998;3(3):169–86.

[6] Freeman MAR, Cameron HU, Brown GC. Cemented double cup arthroplasty of the hip: a 5 year experience with the ICLH prosthesis. Clin Orthop 1978;134: 45–52.

[7] Furaya K, Tsuchiya M, Kawachi S. Socket cup arthroplasty. Clin Orthop 1978;134:41–4.

[8] Howie DW, Campbell D, McGee M, et al. Wagner resurfacing hip arthroplasty. J Bone Joint Surg [Am] 1990;72:708–14.

[9] August AC, Aldam CH, Pynsent PB. The McKee-Farrar hip arthroplasty. A long term study. J Bone Joint Surg [Br] 1986;68:520–7.

[10] Nevelos J, Ahmad Y, Shelton J. Development, validation and multi-centre follow-up of a modern metal-metal hip resurfacing prosthesis [abstract]. Presented at the AAOS Scientific Exhibition, New Orleans, 2003.

[11] Amstutz HC, Campbell PA, Le Duff MJ. Fracture of the neck of the femur after surface arthroplasty of the hip. J Bone Joint Surg [Am] 2004;86(9): 1874–7.

[12] Shimmin AJ, Back DL. Femoral neck fractures associated with hip resurfacing: a national review of 50 cases. J Bone Joint Surg [Br] 2005, in press.

[13] Freeman MAR. Some anatomical and mechanical considerations relevant to the surface replacement of the femoral head. Clin Orthop 1978;134:19–24.

[14] Beaule PE, Lee JL, LeDuff MJ, et al. Orientation of the femoral component in surface arthroplasty of the hip: a biomechanical and clinical analysis. J Bone Joint Surg [Am] 2004;86(9):2015–21.

[15] Campbell P, Mirra H, Amstutz HC. Viability of femoral heads treated with surface arthroplasty. J Arthroplasty 2000;15(1):120–2.

[16] Ganz R, Gill TJ, Guatier E, et al. Surgical dislocation of the adult hip. J Bone Joint Surg [Br] 2001;83(8): 1119–24.

[17] Beaule PE. A soft tissue sparing approach for surface arthroplasty of the hip. Oper Tech Ortho 2004;14(2): 75–84.

[18] Gillespie WJ, Frampton CM, Henderson RJ, et al. The incidence of cancer following total hip replacement. J Bone Joint Surg [Br] 1998;70(4):539–42.

[19] Gillespie WJ, Henry DA, O'Connell DL, et al. Development of haematopoietic cancers after implantation of total joint replacement. Clin Orthop 1996; 329(Suppl):S290–6.

[20] Mathiesen EB, Ahlbom A, Bermann G, et al. Total hip replacement and cancer. A cohort study. J Bone Joint Surg [Br] 1995;77(3):345–50.

[21] Nyren O, McLaughlin JK, Gridley G, et al. Cancer risk after hip replacement with metal implants: a population based cohort study. J Natl Cancer Inst 1995; 87(1):28–33.

[22] Visuri T, Pukkala E, Paavolainen P, et al. Cancer risk after metal on metal and polyethylene on metal total hip arthroplasty. Clin Orthop 1996;329S:S280–9.

[23] Brodner W, Bitzan P, Meisinger V, et al. Elevated serum cobalt with metal on metal articulating surfaces. J Bone Joint Surg [Br] 1997;79(2):316–21.

[24] Jacobs JJ, Skipor AK, Doorn PF, et al. Cobalt and chromium concentrations in patients with metal on metal total hip replacements. Clin Orthop 1996;329S: 256–63.

[25] Maezawa K, Nowaza M, Hirose T, et al. Cobalt and chromium concentrations in patients with metal on metal and other cementless total hip arthroplasty. Arch Orthop Trauma Surg 2002;122(5):283–7.

[26] Skipor AK, Campbell PA, Patterson LM, et al. Serum and urine metal ion levels in patients with metal on metal surface arthroplsty. J Mater Sci Mater Med 2002; 13(12):1227–34.

[27] Back DL, Young DA, Shimmin AJ. Serum metal ion levels following a hip resurfacing. Clin Orthop, in press.

[28] Jacobs JJ, Hallab NJ, Skipor AK, et al. Metal degradation products: a cause for concern in metal-metal bearings? Clin Orthop 2003;417:139–47.

[29] Doorn PF, Mirra JM, Campbell PA, et al. Tissue reaction to metal on metal total hip prestheses. Clin Orthop 1996;329(Suppl):S187–205.

[30] Hallab NJ, Jacobs JJ, Skipor A, et al. Systemic metal-protein binding associated with total joint replacement arthroplasty. J Biomed Mater Res 2000;49(3):353–61.

[31] Hallab NJ, Mikeez K, Jacobs JJ. A triple assay technique for the evaluation of metal induced, delayed type hypersensitivity responses in patients with or receiving total joint arthroplasty. J Biomed Mater Res 2000;53(5):480–9.

[32] Hallab NJ, Merritt K, Jacobs JJ. Metal sensitivity in patients with orthopaedic implants. J Bone Joint Surg [Am] 2001;83:428–36.

[33] Hallab NJ, Mikeez K, Vermes C, et al. Orthopaedic implant related metal toxicity in terms of human lymphocyte reactivity to metal-protein complexes produced from cobalt-base and titanium base implant alloy degradation. Mol Cell Biochem 2001;222(1–2): 127–36.

[34] Urban RM, Jacobs JJ, Tomlinson MJ, et al. Dissemination of wear particles to the liver spleen and abdominal lymph nodes of patients with hip or

knee replacement. J Bone Joint Surg [Am] 2000;82: 457–76.

[35] Clohisy JC, Harris WH. The Harris-Galante porous coated acetabular component with screw fixation. An average ten year follow up study. J Bone Joint Surg [Br] 2004;86(2):177–84.

[36] Kim YH, Kim JS, Cho SH. Primary total hip arthroplasty with a cementless porous coated anatomic total hip prosthesis: 10–12 yr results of prospective and consecutive series. J Arthroplasty 1999;14(5): 538–48.

[37] Ritter MA, Keating EM, Faris PM, et al. Metal-backed acetabular cups in total hip arthroplasty. J Bone Joint Surg [Am] 1990;72(5):672–7.

[38] Ilgen R, Rubash HE. The optimal fixation of the cementless acetabular component in primary total hip arthroplasty. J Am Acad Orthop Surg 2002;10(1): 43–56.

[39] Kienapfel H, Sprey C, Wilke A, et al. Implant fixation by bone ingrowth. J Arthroplasty 1999;14(3):355–68.

[40] Bourne RB, Rorabeck CH, Burkart BC, et al. Ingrowth surfaces. Plasma spray coating to titanium alloy hip replacements. Clin Orthop 1994;298:37–46.

[41] Smith SE, Estok D, Harris WH. Average 12 yr outcome of a chrome–cobalt beaded bony ingrowth acetabular component. J Arthroplasty 1998;13(1):50–60.

[42] Smith SW, Estok DM, Harris WH. Total hip arthroplasty with use of second generation cementing techniques. An eighteen year average follow up study. J Bone Joint Surg [Am] 1998;80(11):1632–40.

[43] Charnley J. The long-term results of low-friction arthroplasty of the hip performed as a primary intervention. J Bone Joint Surg [Br] 1972;54:61–76.

[44] Back DL, Dalziel R, Young DA, et al. Birmingham hip resurfacing: an independent prospective review of 230 hips. J Bone Joint Surg [Br], in press.

ELSEVIER
SAUNDERS

Orthop Clin N Am 36 (2005) 195–201

ORTHOPEDIC
CLINICS
OF NORTH AMERICA

Metal-on-Metal Resurfacing Versus Total Hip Replacement—the Value of a Randomized Clinical Trial

Donald W. Howie, PhD, FRACS, MBBS[a,*], Margaret A. McGee, MPH[a],
Kerry Costi, BA[a], Stephen E. Graves, PhD, FRACS, MBBS[b,c]

[a]Department of Orthopaedics and Trauma, University of Adelaide and Royal Adelaide Hospital, L4 Bice Building,
Adelaide, South Australia 5000, Australia
[b]Department of Medicine, University of Melbourne, Parkville, Victoria 3010, Australia
[c]Department of Orthopaedics, Royal Melbourne Hospital, Parkville, Victoria 3050, Australia

The authors examined the results of resurfacing hip replacement in a randomized clinical trial in patients 55 years of age or younger, comparing metal-on-metal cemented resurfacing hip replacement with cemented total hip replacement. The trial was stopped early because of a high incidence of failure of the cemented resurfacing hip replacement, 8 of 11 hips, mainly caused by failure of the cemented acetabular component, but also because of femoral neck fracture and femoral component loosening that occurred early. Cementless fixation of the acetabular component in resurfacing hip replacement may be an improvement, but no mid to long-term results have been published. Confining resurfacing hip replacement to young patients with good bone and no previous femoral neck surgery may reduce the incidence of early failure. Of significance, there were good results of the cemented collarless double taper femoral stem in young patients after 8–10 years. Although there may be an advantage in bone preservation with resurfacing hip replacement, clinical trials are required to demonstrate it has a midterm success that reasonably approaches that of total hip replacement.

Despite the poor midterm results of metal on polyethylene (m-p) resurfacing hip replacement (RHR) [1–4], interest in RHR remains, particularly for the younger patient, because of the potential for preservation of proximal femoral bone for subsequent revision total hip replacement (THR) [5,6]. New designs of metal-on-metal (m-m) RHR are now available. For these prostheses without demonstrated evidence of clinical effectiveness, comparative clinical evaluation is recommended and should be made available for peer review [7]. Publication enables systematic reviews of results so that the evidence can be compared against benchmarks [8]. Encouraging early-term results for current designs of hybrid m-m RHR recently have been published [9,10]; however, m-m RHR has not been evaluated as part of a randomized clinical trial [8,4,11,12]. Because of these deficiencies in the literature, the aim of this review is to examine the midterm results of a m-m RHR investigated by randomized clinical trial and to propose how RHR should be investigated.

Between October 1993 and August 1995, patients aged 55 years or younger were randomized intraoperatively to receive an m-m cemented RHR or a cemented m-p THR (Table 1). Before randomization, patients who had consented to participate in the trial were stratified by diagnostic group: osteoarthritis or other diagnosis. Randomization of patients within each stratum was undertaken using block randomization techniques with randomly selected block lengths of four or six. Patients with severe osteopo-

This work was supported by the Royal Adelaide Hospital and Corin Baxter Healthcare Pty. Ltd.
* Corresponding author.
E-mail address: donald.howie@adelaide.edu.au
(D.W. Howie).

Table 1
Number of cases, sex ratio, percent osteoarthritis, and median age of cases in the clinical trial

RCT group	n	M:F	% OA	Median age (range) in years
m-m RHR	11	6:5	64%	46 (16–55)
THR	13	9:4	62%	50 (22–54)

Abbreviation: OA, osteoarthritis.

rosis, active infection or those on steroid therapy, bone or systemic diseases associated with poorer outcomes after hip arthroplasty, or medical disorders shortening life expectancy were excluded. The institutional ethics committee approved the trial.

The RHR comprised a low profile McMinn acetabular component and a mini stemmed McMinn femoral resurfacing component (Corin Medical Ltd.; Gloucestershire, UK), both manufactured with high carbon cast cobalt-chrome (Fig. 1A). The nonarticulating surface of the acetabular component was of matte finish and was modified to include recesses to aid cement fixation. The THR comprised an Exeter polished collarless double taper stainless steel femoral stem with a 26-mm diameter steel femoral head and an ultrahigh molecular weight polyethylene acetabular Exeter component (Howmedica Inc.; London, UK) (Fig. 1B).

The arthroplasties were performed by two surgeons (DH and SG) using a posterior approach. One surgeon (DH) undertook all the resurfacing arthroplasties. Patients underwent immediate postoperative weightbearing. Patients underwent regular clinical and radiographic review at 3 and 6 months and at 1 and 2 years and 2–3 yearly thereafter. The trial hypothesis was that when 80% of THR hips have had second femoral revision, less than 50% of RHR hips will have had a second femoral revision. The sample size calculated to achieve sufficient power (0.8) in the study was 47 per group.

Analyses included comparison of postoperative Harris hip and patient derived Harris pain scores [13]

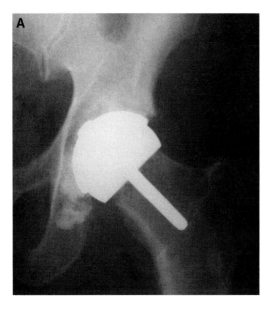
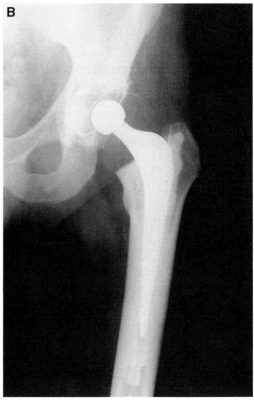

Fig. 1. (*A*) Anteroposterior radiograph of cemented metal–metal resurfacing hip replacement in male patient treated for osteoarthritis of the hip. (*B*) Anteroposterior radiograph of cemented Exeter total hip replacement in male patient treated for osteoarthritis of the hip.

and range of motion. An assessment of cause of failure and component loosening at revision [14] was undertaken also. Assessment of radiographic loosening of the acetabular components was undertaken using the criteria of Hodgkinson et al [15]. Definite radiographic loosening of the femoral THR component was defined as migration of 5 mm or more, excluding subsidence of the stem into the centralizer [12]. Harris' criteria [16] were used to define stable, possibly loose, and probably loose femoral components. Assessment of radiographic loosening of the RHR femoral component was undertaken using the system devised by Amstutz et al [9].

The randomized clinical trial was stopped after 2 years of recruitment because of a high incidence of early failure of the RHR. The primary hypothesis could not be tested. There have been no deaths and no patients lost to follow-up. At latest follow-up (median, 8.5 years; range, 8–10 years), 8 of the 11 (73%) RHRs had been revised to THR. The first three failures of the m-m RHR were caused by femoral neck fractures in two patients and femoral component loosening at the prosthesis–cement and cement–bone interfaces in one patient who had had previous femoral neck surgery (Table 2). Loosening of the cemented metal backed acetabular component was the cause of failure in five cases (Table 2). Loosening was found to have occurred at the prosthesis–cement interface alone in three cases and at the prosthesis–cement and cement–bone interfaces in four cases. Polishing wear of the matte surface of the nonarticulating metal back of the acetabular component was noted commonly at the time of retrieval, confirm-

ing movement of the acetabular component within the cement (Fig. 2). Loosening of the acetabular component in cement also was noted in one of the cases of femoral neck fracture. Osteolytic lesions were evident at the time of revision surgery in the anterior femoral neck in one hip and at the acetabular cement–bone interface in two hips.

Seven of the eight revisions of RHR occurred within 5 years postoperatively. The eighth revision was performed at 9.5 years postoperatively for acetabular component loosening only. The femoral component was solidly fixed. Of the three unrevised RHRs, two acetabular components were radiographically stable (demarcation type 0 and I). The third acetabular component was graded as radiographically unstable because of a gap present at the prosthesis–cement interface in association with a type II demarcation at the cement–bone interface. The femoral components of two of the three unrevised RHRs were radiographically stable with radiolucency scores of 2 and 6 being assigned to the radiographs, respectively. The third femoral component was assigned a radiolucency score of 7, displaying a 0.5-mm incomplete radiolucent line in all three zones of the stem. A pedestal of bone distal to the tip of the stem (zone 2) was evident on the radiographs of each femoral component.

At latest follow-up of the THR group, two cemented acetabular components in two patients had been revised (15%). The reason for revision was loosening at the prosthesis–cement and cement–bone interfaces in one case revised at 5 years, and cement fracture and loosening at the prosthesis–

Table 2
Details of resurfacing hip replacement failures

					Mechanism of failure				
						Loosening grades[a,b]			
						Acetabular component		Femoral component	
Case	Age	Diagnosis	Previous surgery	Months in situ	Fracture neck of femur	p-c	c-b	p-c	c-b
1[c]	53	OA	—	2	✓	2	3 (lysis)	0	0
2	45	OA	—	21	✓	3	0	0	0
3[c]	27	AVN	Fib graft	27	—	3	2	2	3
4	55	OA	—	27	—	3	2	0	0
5	55	OA	—	49	—	3	2	0	0
6	28	AVN	Femoral nail	63	—	3	0	0	0
7	55	OA	—	84	—	3	0	0	0 (lysis)
8	44	OA	—	110	—	2	2	0	0

Abbreviations: AVN, avascular necrosis; OA, osteoarthritis.
[a] Loosening grades: 0, no loosening; 1, fluid movement only at interface; 2, slight movement, requires force such as hammering/leverage to remove; 3, loose, removable by hand.
[b] c-b, cement–bone interface; p-c, prosthesis–cement interface.
[c] Acetabular component revised at subsequent revision procedure.

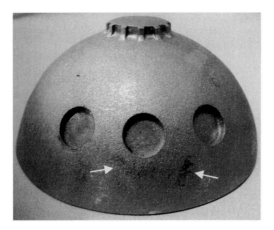

Fig. 2. Retrieved metal resurfacing hip replacement acetabular component with polishing wear (*arrows*) evident on the nonarticulating surface of the component.

cement interface in the other case revised at 9 years. Furthermore, one patient has a radiographically loose acetabular component and is awaiting revision surgery. The remaining eight unrevised acetabular components were radiographically stable with a demarcation type 0 grading. There were no revisions of the polished cemented collarless double taper THR stems and all stems were graded as radiographically stable.

The median Harris hip scores preoperatively were 43/100 and 46/100 for the RHR and THR groups, respectively. Scores improved to 89/100 and 93/100 at 2 years postoperatively for the RHR and THR groups, respectively. The median Harris pain score for patients in the RHR group improved from 10/44 preoperatively to 40/44 at 2 years postoperatively. For patients in the THR group, the median preoperative Harris pain score was 20/44, and this improved to 44/44 at 2 years postoperatively (Fig. 3). The range of motion of the operated hip joint, defined as flexion range or abduction to adduction or rotation, were comparable between groups at up to 2 years postoperatively (Table 3).

There have been no other published articles to date that investigate the outcomes of new generation RHR versus THR as part of a randomized clinical trial. This trial in young patients was stopped early because of a high failure rate of the RHR, and particularly of the acetabular component.

Early designs of m-p RHRs had high failure rates because of acetabular wear and loosening and a small incidence of early femoral failure caused by femoral neck fractures and component loosening [2,4,17–19]. These problems were attributed to design and surgical and patient related factors. The larger diameter of these RHRs required a thin polyethylene acetabular component that suffered from loosening, wear, and impingement wear. Subsequent RHR prostheses were

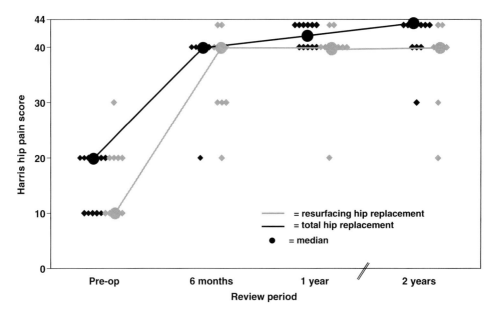

Fig. 3. Early Harris hip pain scores for patients treated with resurfacing hip replacement and patients treated with total hip replacement.

Table 3
Range of motion of hip following hip replacement

Range of motion parameter	Group	Range of motion in degrees—median (range)[a] by follow-up period			
		3 months	6 months	1 year	2 years
Flexion range	RHR	90 (50–120)	90 (70–130)	95 (75–115)	110 (60–120)
		90 (50–120)	*85 (70–130)*	*95 (75–115)*	*105 (60–120)*
	THR	90 (70–100)	90 (70–110)	100 (80–120)	105 (80–120)
Abduction to adduction	RHR	50 (20–60)	60 (40–80)	60 (50–90)	70 (30–80)
		50 (20–60)	*55 (40–80)*	*60 (50–90)*	*73 (30–80)*
	THR	45 (30–75)	50 (30–90)	55 (40–85)	50 (30–90)
Rotation in extension	RHR	35 (15–70)	50 (30–75)	55 (30–105)	40 (10–60)
		35 (15–70)	*50 (40–50)*	*55 (30–70)*	*40 (10–50)*
	THR	35 (10–60)	50 (30–75)	55 (35–90)	50 (30–70)
Rotation at 60° flexion	RHR	35 (0–50)	50 (20–105)	55 (30–85)	60 (10–85)
		35 (0–50)	*50 (30–60)*	*60 (30–85)*	*60 (10–85)*
	THR	30 (0–65)	40 (10–105)	50 (20–75)	45 (30–65)

Abbreviations: RHR, resurfacing hip replacement; THR, total hip replacement.
 [a] Results in italics, excludes RHR cases revised within 4 years.

modified and cemented and cementless metal–metal articulations were introduced in the 1990s. Results of these designs have been reported [20–22], but the follow-up periods were short.

Two of the early failures of the m-m RHR were caused by femoral neck fracture in a 53-year-old patient and a 45-year-old patient, and in both patients notching of the neck was not seen at surgery. These failures, and the case of femoral loosening, reinforce the opinion that RHR should be confined to young patients who have good bone [9] and who have had no previous femoral neck surgery.

The loosening of the acetabular component raises some issues. Loosening may have been caused by the design, which was a stiff metal component that relied on recesses and a small protrusion in the back of the component for cement interdigitation. Although cemented fixation of the m-m RHR acetabular component is no longer used, there remains concern that a large diameter metal-on-metal articulation may predispose to increased strain at the implant–bone interface and increase the friction torque to a level greater than that consistent with long-term fixation of the acetabular component. New designs of m-m RHR have a porous coated cementless acetabular component that eliminates the potential for loosening of the acetabular component in the cement [9,10]. It is likely that cementless fixation of the acetabular component is an improvement, and recent results of current designs of m-m RHR at an average follow-up of 3.5 years [9] and 3.3 years [10] are excellent. Longer-term follow-up of these studies and results from less experienced surgeons not involved in the design of these prostheses are necessary to demonstrate

that cementless acetabular fixation for m-m RHR is successful.

An important finding in this study was the failure of two cemented acetabular components of the THR in this young cohort. One component was revised for loosening and another for cement fracture and a further case is awaiting revision surgery. Of clinical significance in this randomized clinical trial is that the cemented collarless double taper femoral stem of the Exeter design has performed well at midterm follow-up. Furthermore, it has been claimed that RHR gives better range of motion of the hip than does THR. The authors found no differences in the range of flexion or rotation between groups. With regard to abduction–adduction range of motion, there was no difference between the ranges of values, and the difference in the median values was considered unimportant given the small number of patients in each group.

The place for RHR would best be determined by way of randomized clinical trials to demonstrate it is as good as or better than primary THR, which now has good mid- to long-term results in young patients [23–25]. Large sample sizes are needed to demonstrate that RHR is better than THR and multicenter trials are necessary to achieve these sample sizes in young patients. Sensitive outcomes instruments, including radiostereometric analysis to assess early fixation and biologic monitoring of metal levels in patients with m-m RHR [11], are important.

Although patients in this trial provided samples of blood and urine for the purpose of biologic monitoring for metal levels, these analyses were not undertaken because of the high incidence of early acetabular component loosening at the prosthesis–

cement interface and resultant wear of the metal acetabular component, making results difficult to interpret. Nevertheless, the authors emphasize the importance of comparing levels in patients with clinically successful m-m hip replacement with those in patients with traditional m-p articulations.

The previous earlier designs of RHR using an m-p articulation were poor. Before this was recognized, however, resurfacings had been used in large numbers of patients, many of whom underwent unnecessarily early revision surgery. In contrast, the current randomized clinical trial demonstrated how sensitive such a trial is in detecting early failure caused by an inadequate prosthesis design, supporting the concept of stepwise introduction of technology [26]. The safety and efficacy of this design of resurfacing was assessed rapidly before being used in a large cohort of patients, which disproves the claim that randomized clinical trials do not act as an early warning system for implants that fail prematurely [27].

Compared with comparative cohort studies, randomized clinical trials remain the best level of evidence when evaluating the outcomes of different interventions [28,29]. Of significance, in randomized clinical trials, pretreatment stratification of patients increases the likelihood that known and unknown prognostic factors are distributed equally across both groups, thus reducing the effects of confounders on outcome. Furthermore, the conduct of trials increases the likelihood that patients are followed well, using comprehensive outcome parameters, and that loss to follow-up is kept to a minimum, the latter being a common problem in prospective cohort series. The limitations of randomized clinical trials are well known. These include their costs and the applicability of findings when manufacturers continue to redesign joint replacement implants under study. Good results of randomized clinical trials, which often are conducted in tertiary referral hospitals, are also no guarantee of the absence of problems once prostheses are used widely in the community [30], thus highlighting the importance of post-marketing surveillance systems. Because randomized clinical trials have well defined inclusion and exclusion criteria, however, the generalizability of the findings to the general population are known early.

Summary

In summary, resurfacing hip replacement is an appealing option for bone preservation in the younger patient. In the current study of a metal-on-metal resurfacing design, cemented fixation of the acetabular component was inadequate. Although this may be design related, the early failures, including some on the femoral side, raise concern about the potentially deleterious effects of a large articulation and possibly increased frictional torque. These findings emphasize the importance of randomized clinical trials in evaluating this type of new technology.

Acknowledgments

The authors thank Scott Brumby, Susan Pannach, and Professor Robert Bauze for their contribution to the study.

References

[1] Amstutz HC, Graff-Radford A, Mai LL, Thomas BJ. Surface replacements of the hip with the Tharies system: two- to five-year results. Clin Orthop 1981; 63:1069–77.

[2] Cotella L, Railton GT, Nunn D, Freeman MAR, Revell PA. ICLH double-cup arthroplasty, 1980–1987. J Arth 1990;5:349–57.

[3] Freeman MAR, Cameron HU, Brown GC. Cemented double cup arthroplasty of the hip: a 5-year experience with the ICLH prosthesis. Clin Orthop 1978;134: 45–53.

[4] Trentani C, Vaccarino FP. Complications in surface replacement arthroplasty of the hip: experience with the Paltrinieri-Trentani prosthesis. Int Orthop 1981; 4:247–52.

[5] Kim WC, Grogan T, Amstutz HC, Dorey F. Survivorship comparison of Tharies and conventional hip arthroplasty in patients younger than 40 years old. Clin Orthop 1987;214:269–77.

[6] Wagner H. Surface replacement arthroplasty of the hip. Clin Orthop 1978;134:36–40.

[7] National Institute for Clinical Excellence (NICE). Guidance on the selection of prostheses for primary total hip replacement. London: NICE; 2000.

[8] Moher D, Schulz KF, Altman DG. The Consort statement: revised recommendations for improving the quality of reports of parallel-group randomised trials. Lancet 2001;357:1191–4.

[9] Amstutz HC, Beaulé PE, Dorey FJ, Le Duff MJ, Campbell PA, Gruen TA. Metal-on-metal hybrid surface arthroplasty: two- to six-year follow-up study. J Bone Joint Surg 2004;86A:28–39.

[10] Daniel J, Pynsent PB, McMinn DJW. Metal-on-metal resurfacing of the hip in patients under the age of 55 years with osteoarthritis. J Bone Joint Surg 2004; 86B:177–83.

[11] Amstutz HC, Campbell P, McKellop H, et al. Metal on

metal total hip replacement workshop consensus document. Clin Orthop 1996;329S:297–303.

[12] Malchau H, Karrholm J, Wang YX, Herberts P. Accuracy of migration analysis in hip arthroplasty. Digitized and conventional radiography, compared to radiostereometry in 51 patients. Acta Orthop Scand 1995;66:418–24.

[13] Harris WH. Traumatic arthritis of the hip after dislocation and acetabular fractures: treatment by mold arthroplasty. J Bone Joint Surg 1969;51A:737–55.

[14] Howie DW, Cornish BL, Vernon-Roberts B. Resurfacing hip arthroplasty. Classification of loosening and the role of prosthesis wear particles. Clin Orthop 1990; 255:144–59.

[15] Hodgkinson JP, Shelley P, Wroblewski BM. The correlation between the roentgenographic appearance and operative findings at the bone–cement junction of the socket in Charnley low friction arthroplasties. Clin Orthop 1988;228:105–9.

[16] Harris WH, McCarthey JC, O'Neill DA. Femoral component loosening using contemporary techniques of femoral cement fixation. J Bone Joint Surg 1982; 64A:1063–7.

[17] Amstutz HC, Dorey F, O'Carroll PF. Tharies resurfacing arthroplasty. Evolution and long-term results. Clin Orthop 1986;213:92–114.

[18] Franzen H, Mjoberg B, Rydholm U. Metal backing improves the survival of surface replacement of the hip. Arch Orthop Trauma Surg 1993;112:257–9.

[19] Howie DW, Campbell DC, McGee M, Cornish BL. Wagner resurfacing hip arthroplasty. J Bone Joint Surg 1990;72A:708–14.

[20] McMinn D, Treacy R, Lin K, Pynsent P. Metal on metal surface replacement of the hip. Experience of the McMinn prosthesis. Clin Orthop 1996;329S:89–98.

[21] Schmalzreid TP, Fowble VA, Ure KJ, Amstutz HC. Metal on metal surface replacement of the hip. Technique, fixation and early results. Clin Orthop 1996;329S:106–14.

[22] Wagner M, Wagner H. Preliminary results of uncemented metal on metal stemmed and resurfacing hip replacement arthroplasty. Clin Orthop 1996;329S: 78–88.

[23] Malchau H, Herberts P, Eisler T, Garellick G, Soderman P. The Swedish total hip replacement register. J Bone Joint Surg 2002;84A:2–20.

[24] Smith SE, Estock Jr DM, Harris WH. 20-year experience with cemented primary and conversion total hip arthroplasty using so-called second-generation cementing techniques in patients aged 50 years or younger. J Arth 2000;15:263–73.

[25] Sochart DH, Porter ML. The long-term results of Charnley low-friction arthroplasty in young patients who have congenital dislocation, degenerative osteoarthrosis, or rheumatoid arthritis. J Bone Joint Surg 1997;79:1599–617.

[26] Malchau H. On the importance of stepwise introduction of new hip implant technology [thesis]. Göteberg, Sweden: Göteberg University; 1995.

[27] Bourne RB, Maloney WJ, Wright JG. An AOA critical issue. The outcome of the outcomes movement. J Bone Joint Surg 2004;86A:633–40.

[28] The Cochrane Collaboration. Available at: www.cochrane.org. Accessed July 2004.

[29] Laupacis A, Rorabeck CH, Bourne RB, et al. Randomised trials in orthopaedics: why, how and when? J Bone Joint Surg 1989;71A:535–43.

[30] Bunker JP. Is efficiency the gold standard for quality assessment. Inq 1988;25:51–8.

ELSEVIER
SAUNDERS

Orthop Clin N Am 36 (2005) 203 – 213

ORTHOPEDIC
CLINICS
OF NORTH AMERICA

Belgium Experience with Metal-on-Metal Surface Arthroplasty

Koen A. De Smet, MD[a,b,*]

[a]Hipcentre, Jan Palfijn Hospital, Henri Dunantlaan 5, B-9000 Ghent, Belgium
[b]Anca Clinic, Kalverbosstraat 31 A, B-9070 Heusden, Belgium

Metal-on-metal resurfacing is increasingly becoming widely used. The history of failures with the Charnley teflon-on-teflon and the Wagner/Tharies metal-on-polyethylene prostheses makes resurfacing controversial [1–6]. Results achieved with the new metal-on-metal resurfacing are starting to be published [7–15].

With the introduction of a metal-on-metal resurfacing prosthesis and a refined instrumentation, high volumetric polyethylene wear and malpositioning of the head component on the femoral neck—problems encountered with earlier designs—should be avoided [16–18].

The short-term clinical results are excellent; none of the early problems associated with the metal-on-polyethylene resurfacing have been encountered [9,11,15].

Theoretic advantages are less bone destruction, less bone resection, normal femoral loading, avoidance of stress shielding, maximum proprioceptive feedback, and restoration of normal anatomy. In addition, reduced risk of dislocation, less leg inequality problems, and easier revision should convince surgeons to favor metal-on-metal resurfacing. When infection occurs, a one-stage revision and a smaller contamination is likely.

The purpose of this study is to review the early clinical results of a hybrid metal-on-metal surface arthroplasty and analyze the clinical outcome, level of activity, and radiologic findings. A first Belgian experience with a well-documented prospective series is presented.

Materials and methods

From September 1998 to April 2004, 1114 metal-on-metal resurfacings were performed by the author. Most implants were Birmingham Hip Resurfacings (BHR; Midland Medical Technologies, Birmingham UK; Smith and Nephew, Memphis, Tennessee); the Conserve Plus (Wright Medical, Arlington, Tennessee) was used in 20 cases and the Durom (Zimmer, Wintherthur, Switzerland) device was used in 6 cases. This article presents a consecutive series of the first 252 patients (all BHR) with a clinical follow-up from 2 to 5 years. Patients were clinically scored with the Harris Hip and Postel Merle d'Aubigné scores, hip range of movement, and activity. Follow-up was done at 6 weeks, 6 months, 1 year, and then at 1- or 2-year intervals. Data were collected intraoperatively and postoperatively in a prospective way. Data storage and processing was done using the Orthowave and Statwave software (ARIA-GreyStone, Bruay Labuissiere, France).

Age at surgery ranged from 16 to 75 years, with a mean of 49.7 years. The mean weight was 81.9 kg (range, 44–140 kg; SD, 16). Body mass index averaged 27.1 (range, 18.8–47.9; SD, 4.3). Left and right hip distribution was equal (52.9 and 47.1, respectively). More male patients (68.9%) were treated than female patients (31.1%) (Table 1). The percentage of patients in Charnley group A was 93.8%, the

---

* Anca Clinic, Kalverbosstraat 31 A, B-9070 Heusden, Belgium.
E-mail address: koen.desmet@skynet.be

Table 1
Sex and age of patients

Patients	Number	Mean age (y)	Range
Total	252	49.7	16–75
Male	176	49.6	17–75
Female	76	50.1	16–69

percentage in group B was 3.1%, and in group C, 3.1% [19].

Sixteen cases were bilateral resurfacings. In 237 cases, a normal BHR was used; in 15 cases, a BHR with dysplasia cup was used (Fig. 1). The mean length of hospital stay was 7 days (range, 2–25 days; SD, 3.5).

Indications

The author's institution has almost no contra-indications for hip resurfacing arthroplasty. No avascular necrosis (even with severe femoral bone loss) (Fig. 2) or rheumatoid arthritis was excluded. An age limit was set to 65 years for male patients and to 60 years for female patients. Patients older than this limit who had a high activity level (UCLA activity scale >7) and good bone quality on radiograph (fluted champagne glass–shaped femur, thick femoral cortex, and good trabecular structure in the femoral neck) were also included. Preoperative diagnoses are shown in Table 2.

The only exclusion criterion was a too-deformed femoral head, whereby offset and leg length could not be restored with a resurfacing procedure.

Preoperative scores were not collected because no patients received an arthroplasty when the Harris Hip Score was higher than 60.

Radiographic follow-up

All radiographs were evaluated immediately postoperatively and at 6 weeks, 1 year, 2 years, and at the latest follow-up. Osteolysis, reactive and radiolucent lines, heterotopic ossification, bone remodeling, development of cysts, migration of the components, bone resorption or narrowing at the femoral neck, and lines around screws (dysplasia cups) were noted [11,20,21]. In the first 115 prostheses, several angles were measured on the preoperative and postoperative radiographs and registered (measurement on digitalized radiographs, standing pelvis, Siemens Endomap). Five measurements were done to evaluate the reproducibility of placement of the BHR prosthesis. The preoperative angle of the femoral neck was measured (Fig. 3). The postoperative angle of the head of the prosthesis was measured in relation to the shaft of the femur. The obtained result and the difference with the preoperative neck-shaft angle were determined. The abduction angle of the acetabular component was measured, and parallelism with the femoral component was noted [9].

Operative technique

All surgeries were performed through an extended standard posterior approach. The maximus split extends about 10 to 15 cm into the muscle. The insertion of the gluteus maximus tendon is fully released to allow easy anterior displacement of the femur and femoral head to perform the acetabular procedure. The gluteus maximus tendon is released with cauterization close to the bone. The tendon is never reattached for risk of entrapment of the sciatic nerve in the suture. Exposure is never jeopardized by

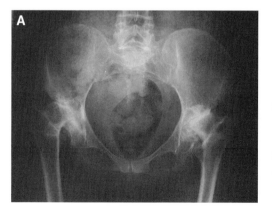
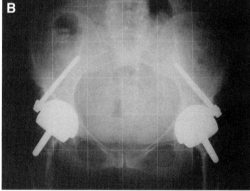

Fig. 1. Bilateral dysplasia BHR. (*A*) Preoperative x-ray. (*B*) Postoperative x-ray at 3 years.

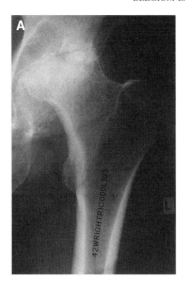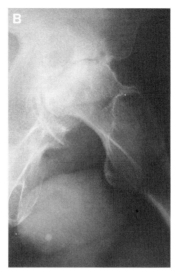

Fig. 2. Avascular necrosis (Ficat IV). (*A*) Anteroposterior view. (*B*) Lateral view.

a smaller or minimal incision. The capsule is divided circumferentially near the border of the acetabulum (1 cm). The posterior part of the capsule is incised as posterior as possible to not damage the soft tissue of the femoral neck. The circumflex vessels are always coagulated and divided. The soft tissues around the femoral neck are kept completely intact, and the capsule is not removed. Acetabular reaming is done as in a normal total hip procedure. A cup position of no more than 45° of abduction and an anatomic anteversion of 20° to 30° are aimed for.

Less anteversion can result in groin pain from local conflict with anterior structures and the psoas tendon. All resurfacing devices are chrome/cobalt alloys, which are stiffer implants than the more often used uncemented total hip titanium alloy cups. Therefore, a bigger force is needed to impact the cup. The absence of holes in the cup to see if it is fully seated explains the need for a hammer of at least 1 kg. In the BHR system, there is a possible additional screw fixation using a dysplasia device with two specially threaded screws. This cup only finds its application in congenital dislocation or severe developmental dysplasia in which a press-fit with a normal cup cannot be obtained. The superolateral aspect is grafted with autologous grafts from the reaming of the head and cup.

On the femoral side, meticulous placement of the central pin in the middle of the femoral neck is

Table 2
Etiology (N = 252)

Preoperative diagnosis	Indications	
	n	%
Osteoarthritis	203	80.56
Necrosis	22	7.26
Congenital dislocation of the hip	12	4.76
Rheumatoid	9	3.57
Traumatic	3	1.19
Neurometabolic	1	0.4
Other	2	0.79

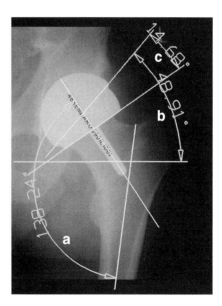

Fig. 3. Postoperative measurements. a, postoperative angle of the head of the prosthesis in relation to the shaft of the femur; b, abduction angle of the acetabular component; c, parallelism with the femoral component.

of capital importance. In addition, the varus-valgus angle and anteversion should be checked at the same time. A lateral femoral guide pin in the BHR system is helpful but can be forgotten at the end of surgery. In the other resurfacing systems, the varus-valgus angle and anteversion is assessed by eye. A goniometric device can help find a more correct varus-valgus angulation. In all cases, a 140° angle position is aimed for. Eight to 10 cement fixation holes of 4 to 5 mm are made before cementing the head component. When the bone is sclerotic, more and smaller holes (2 mm) are drilled (Fig. 4).

A femoral suction device is inserted into the lesser trochanter and keeps the femoral head dry and clean for cementing. It is inserted at the beginning of the femoral procedure. It also prevents general embolism and local thrombogenesis. Two-thirds of the head component is filled with tobramycin antibiotic cement (Surgical Simplex; Stryker, Mahwah, New Jersey) and impacted at 1 minute, 15 seconds. Before impaction, the femoral head is always pulse lavaged to clear the spongious bone. In large femoral defects (avascular necrosis), a longer time is waited (up to 2 minutes) to apply the head component. In avascular necrosis, all of the dead bone is removed and no bone grafts are used. Even in severe femoral bone deficiency in avascular necrosis, resurfacing is done. As long as there is a circumferential seal at the head-neck junction of the femur for the head component, cement pressurization can be obtained and resurfacing is not contraindicated.

Minimal bone resection is obtained with a size-to-size (line-to-line) placement of the femoral component on the bone. A line-to-line technique enhances a good primary fit, stability, and fixation. The impaction of the BHR femoral head sometimes requires a great deal of force because of a tight fit without cement extrusion. Marking the exact edge of the prosthesis on the femoral head-neck junction, before impaction, also helps to place the head implant at the

---

Box 1. Risk factors for femoral neck fracture

Notching the neck of the femur (cutting with cylindric reamer into the cortex of the femoral neck)
Malpositioning of the central guide pin
Varus placement of the head component
Incomplete coverage of the reamed bone
Removing soft tissues around the femoral neck (making the neck avascular)
Impacting too hard and too long
Too much cement in the implant
Waiting too long before starting to impact
Not marking the end position of the implant before impaction
Impacting in the wrong direction
Removing too much bone of the femoral neck (head component too small)
Severe osteoporosis

---

ideal position and stop the impaction at the right time (Box 1). Proper preoperative templating is very important and the first indicator for the size of implant to be used.

Thorough covering and draping of soft tissues and muscles before the preparation of the femoral head and the use of pulse lavage reduces heterotopic bone formation.

In the first 900 cases, a tight closure of all posterior structures, external rotators, and the trochanteric bursa was done. In the cases that followed, only the posterior capsule and piriformis tendon were reattached.

Postoperative protocol

Prophylactic cephazolin was administered for 18 hours (3 doses of 2 g). The patients were placed on low molecular weight subcutaneous heparins (nadroparine) for 3 weeks starting the day before surgery. In every patient, prophylactic indomethacin was given for 3 weeks (3 doses of 25 mg daily). In risk patients (ankylosing spondylitis, post-traumatic cases), a single irradiation dose of 7 Gy was given.

Patients were mobilized on the first postoperative day and allowed immediate full weight bearing. The average length of stay was 5 days, with discharge home on the third day post surgery. Patients were not given any further restrictions in activity. Patients

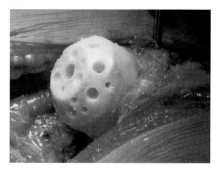

Fig. 4. Big and smaller cement fixation holes.

Table 3
Problems and risks encountered in sizing the resurfacing implant

Acetabular component	Femoral component
Too big	
Leg lengthening	Leg lengthening
Not covering implant and local conflict	Not covering implant and local conflict
Too much bone removal	
Malpositioning	
Loss of press-fit	
Too small	
No problems	Leg shortening
	Higher risk of notching and fracture
	Higher risk of avascular necrosis and stress fracture
	Risk of impingement
	Higher risk of dislocation

used two crutches for 10 to 14 days and then one crutch for another 2 weeks.

Component sizing

Choosing the right component size is often difficult. In resurfacing, there often is the choice of more bone removal from the acetabulum or from the femur. To adapt the cup to a big enough head size on the femur, a larger sized cup than might normally be selected is used. The choice is better range of motion with a bigger head size, bigger cup, and more acetabular bone removal or the possibility of impingement and less mobility in flexion with a smaller head size, smaller cup, and more acetabular bone preservation (Table 3).

Results

Clinical results

The duration of follow-up is from 2 to 5 years, with a mean for the group of 2.8 years. Of the 252 first patients, only 3 (four prostheses) were lost to further follow-up because they died. At the most recent follow-up, 97.8% had no pain. The total Harris Hip Score averaged 97.24 (range, 41–100; SD, 7.6). The mean Postel Merle d'Aubigné score was 17.68 (range, 12–18; SD, 0.9). Sixty-one percent of the patients performed strenuous activities (strenuous, 60.53%; activities of daily living, 38.60%; independent, 0.88%). Hip flexion averaged 123° (range, 50°–145°; SD, 13) (Table 4). There was no clear

clinical evidence of leg lengthening (mean, 0.07 cm) in the overall group.

Forty-nine patients (19.4%) experienced a clicking, clocking, or clunking noise or feeling in the prosthesis that occurred in the first 6 months after surgery but was painless and disappeared progressively.

In 1.2% (3/252) of patients, squeaking noises appeared in the 2-year period after surgery. The duration of the noise was less than 24 hours and a one-time incidence. The noise started when the patient had an increase or change in activities. Stair climbing always generated or increased the noise. The sound was similar to a nonlubricated creaking door hinge.

Seven patients (2.8%) had a persistent slight groin pain. Four patients (1.6%) had no adverse effects with activity, but three patients could not do impact sports because of this problem and had to reduce their activity level (UCLA activity <8).

Radiographic results

Preoperative and postoperative measurements were done on 115 resurfacings. A slight valgus placement of the head component is aimed for. A 140° positioning seems to be a good position for force transfer to the bone, femoral head, and neck. The mean preoperative angle of the femoral neck was 134.9° (range, 113°–148°; SD, 6.8). The obtained mean postoperative angle of the femoral head component was 137.6° degrees (range, 125°–156°; SD, 5.9).

In the full series (252 patients), osteolysis, reactive lines, migration of a component, or neck narrowing was seen in only two revision cases.

In the avascular necrosis case, a radiolucent line was seen in Amstutz et al's [11] "peg zone." The stem of the prosthesis moved progressively away from this line, indicating a loosening of the femoral component (Fig. 5). In the low-grade infection case, an osteolytic line in the three peg zones around the femoral stem and a progressive acetabular osteolysis were seen. There was also neck narrowing (Fig. 6).

Table 4
Harris Hip Score, Postel Merle d'Aubigné score, and flexion at follow-up

Measures	Median	Range	SD
HHS	97.24	41–100	7.6
PMA	17.68	12–18	0.9
Flexion	123°	50°–145°	13

Abbreviations: HHS, Harris Hip Score; PMA, Postel Merle d'Aubigné score.

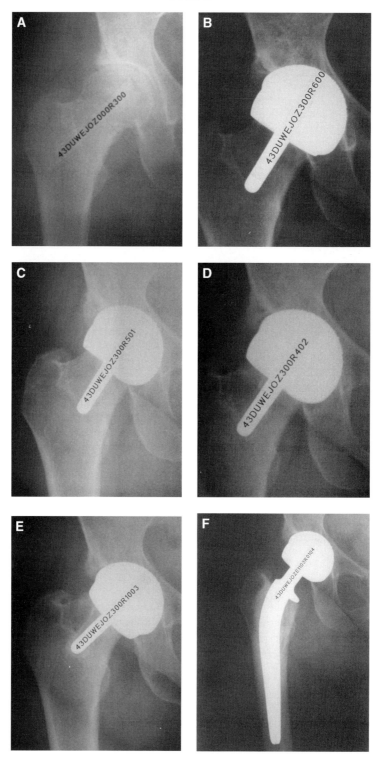

Fig. 5. Radiographs showing avascular necrosis of the head. (*A*) Preoperative. (*B*) Nine months postoperative. (*C*) One year postoperative. (*D*) Two years postoperative. (*E*) Three years postoperative. (*F*) Revision. Note the changing reactive line at the metaphyseal stem of the prosthesis (Amstutz et al's [11] peg zone 1).

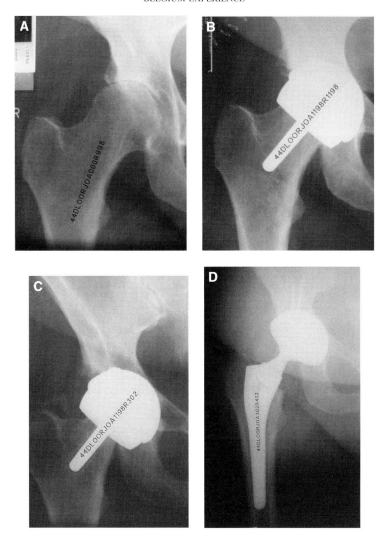

Fig. 6. Radiographs showing low-grade infection. In addition to osteolysis in all cup zones and the femoral neck, an osteolytic line is seen in the three zones around the stem. (*A*) Preoperative. (*B*) Immediate postoperative. (*C*) Four years postoperative. (*D*) Revision.

The diagnosis was made by anatomopathology and a possible *Staphyloccus aureus* specimen was identified on enriched cultures.

At the latest follow-up, all reviewed radiographs showed no bone resorption or osteolysis. No loosening of head or cup components was seen. Impingement of the neck can lead to remodeling the shape of the femoral neck (Fig. 7).

Complications

A summary of the complications is listed in Table 5. Both cases of sciatic nerve palsies with drop foot showed no evidence of recovery at the latest follow-up, which was more than 2 years postsurgery. In one case, a guide pin was inadvertently left in situ. The pin was not removed, and is still in place 4 years later. The postoperative deep venous thrombosis and pulmonary embolism cases were treated with anticoagulants with no further problems. Four cases of heterotopic ossification were seen: three Brooker grade 1 and one Brooker grade 2. There was no functional impairment in these cases. There were two dislocations in the same patient (4 months and 1 year post surgery). The dislocations were traumatic (fall) and occurred twice in an inebriated male patient; reduction was done without anesthesia.

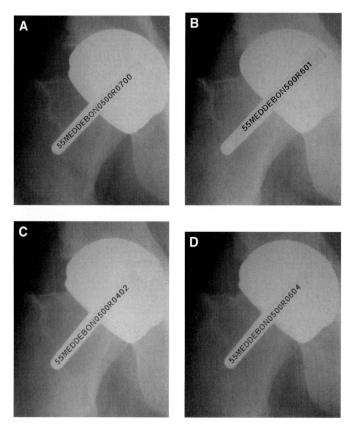

Fig. 7. Remodeling of the proximal lateral femoral neck at (*A*) 2 months, (*B*) 1 year, (*C*) 2 years, and (*D*) 4.5 years after surgery.

Failures

Three failures needed revision or reoperation (Table 6). The femoral neck fracture case occurred 3 weeks after surgery in a 42-year-old male patient with cerebral palsy and muscular spasticity. A difficult reduction in this developmental hip dysplasia case and osteoporosis could have led to an intra-

operative stress fracture of the femoral neck. A reoperation was done with a modular head on a cemented stem.

The avascular necrosis case was treated before fracture at 3 years, 7 months. Radiographic changes were noted at the 2-year follow-up period (but retrospectively, changes could be seen the 1-year follow-up; see Fig. 5). Diagnosis was done by bone scintigraphy (no vascularity of the femoral head in the blood pool phase). The patient had a postoperative stem-shaft angle of the head component of 139°, a UCLA activity level of 6, weight of 57 kg, no previous surgery, and no cyst bigger than 1 cm, which means that the patient had a Surface Arthroplasty Risk Index [12] of 2. For revision, a cemented stem with a modular head was used without changing the cup. The patient had a full recovery and increased satisfaction compared with the first surgery.

The low-grade infection case was first seen on radiograph after the 2-year follow-up. Diagnosis was done by bone scan, white blood cell scan, bone marrow scan, and was confirmed by anatomopathology.

Table 5
Complications in metal-on-metal resurfacing (11/252)

Complications	n	%
Sciatic nerve palsy with drop foot (no recovery >2 y)	2	0.8
Pin in femur	1	0.4
Deep venous thrombosis	1	0.4
Pulmonary embolism	1	0.4
Heterotopic ossification Brooker grade 1	3	1.2
Heterotopic ossification Brooker grade 2	1	0.4
Dislocation (not recurrent)	1	0.4
Infection	1	0.4

Table 6
Failures, time to failure, and type of surgery

Failures	n	Time to failure	Type of surgery
Femoral neck fracture	1	3 wk	Cemented stem + modular head
Avascular necrosis of the femoral head	1	2 y	Cemented stem + modular head
Low-grade infection	1	2 y	Cleaning and exchange to primary uncemented total hip arthroplasty

The patient had a postoperative stem-shaft angle of 136°, a UCLA activity level of 4, weight of 97 kg, no previous surgery, and no cyst bigger than 1 cm (Surface Arthroplasty Risk Index = 0). Revision took place at 3 years, 4 months (see Fig. 3) and was treated as a one-stage procedure; a primary ceramic-on-ceramic uncemented total hip prosthesis was implanted. There was no femoral loosening.

Discussion

The early clinical and radiologic results in this group of metal-on-metal resurfacings are satisfactory, with Harris Hip and Postel Merle d'Aubigné scores indicating early clinical success. The high percentage of strenuous activity (61%) in this young patient group satisfies the expectations of the hip resurfacing procedure; notably, anatomic restoration with restoration of leg length and offset. The large diameter of the resurfacing is the reason for the low dislocation rate (0.4%).

Clinical perceptions in patients such as a squeaking noise or clicking or clunking noises and feelings in the prosthesis are new features in hip resurfacing. The clicking and clunking noises and feelings in the first 6 months after surgery are a possible temporary decoaptation of both components; they are painless and subside after the capsule and muscles around the hip are fully healed. The squeaking noises are possibly produced due to a temporary lack of lubrication—a dry running of the metal-on-metal prosthesis. It did not occur after 2 years, an interval that equals the running-in period of a metal-on-metal friction couple. The understanding of this benign incident can prevent misunderstanding and panic in patients and orthopedic surgeons.

Only further follow-up can tell whether these noises and feelings will result in a poor later outcome. Groin pain—the result of repetitive trauma to the femoral neck and soft tissues and structures around it or local conflict with tendons and muscles—can be explained by too little anteversion of the cup, the selection of an acetabular implant that is too big, or a femoral component that is malpositioned or too big. A femoral component that is too small or tighter to the femoral neck results in less flexion and possible impingement. Higher activity levels or participation in impact sports can be jeopardized because of this groin problem. Clinical examination gives the diagnosis of femoral neck conflict, with pain in the groin when the hip is flexed more than 90° in neutral abduction and with endorotation of the limb. When the leg is abducted with the same movements, the

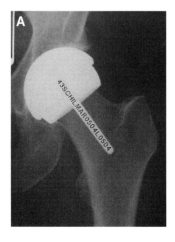
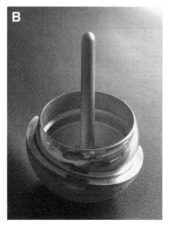

Fig. 8. (*A*) Conserve Plus Thin Shell x-ray, anteroposterior view. (*B*) Implant.

conflict with the femoral neck will be by-passed. A rubbing psoas or hip flexor tendon will give groin pain on active raising of the straight leg. A local anesthetic infiltration will also diagnose this problem.

The 4-mm implant-size increments with the BHR system lead to a higher risk in potentially oversizing the cup with the noted problems. With the polyethylene and cable impactor system, the BHR cup placement becomes technically demanding. An implant with 2-mm increments and a thin shell cup gives a lower risk for these problems. Two-millimeter implant-size increments also result in a smaller risk of oversizing or undersizing of the implant. For this reason, manufacturers today produce thinner acetabular implants. A lower-profile impactor, such as used with the Conserve Plus Thin Shell (Wright Medical) design (Fig. 8), gives a better control of the anteversion during insertion of the device. A better range of movement should be achieved with a larger head size, but it depends on the head-to-neck ratio, the existence of osteophytes, and the positioning of the implants.

Proper anteversion in the cup and meticulous removal of all osteophytes are important. The anterior femoral neck often needs reshaping. As stated earlier, the choice is better range of motion with a bigger head size, bigger cup, and more acetabular bone removal or the possibility of impingement and less mobility in flexion with a smaller head size, smaller cup, and more acetabular bone preservation. In the author's experience, line-to-line placement of the femoral head component (without cement mantle), multiple fixation holes, and a cementing technique with pressurization and pulse lavage are necessary to get an optimal fixation of the implant.

As of the latest follow-up in this series, no adverse effect was seen in the more varus placement of the head components as has been seen in other series [11].

Cementing of the stem is not advised by the author because stress distribution by the stem is not desirable, and the first signs on radiographs (femoral loosening, avascular necrosis, infection, wear), which are often seen around the stem of the resurfacing, may be masked. Long-term follow-up is needed to see whether varus placement has an adverse effect on the fixation and loosening of the head as was stated in the Amstutz et al series [11].

Using exclusively alternate bearings in patients under the age of 75 years, metal-on-metal resurfacing appears to be a good alternative in young active patients. The short-term results are promising. Meticulous surgical technique and planning are the key factors to an excellent postoperative result.

Reproducible placement of the prosthesis components should be possible and the wear properties of metal-on-metal should guarantee a good long-term follow-up. Time will tell whether this target can be achieved.

References

[1] Freeman MAR, Cameron HU, Brown GC. Cemented double-cup arthroplasty of the hip. A 5 year experience with the ICLH prosthesis. Clin Orthop 1978; 134:45–52.

[2] Furuya K, Tsuchiya M, Kawachi S. Socket cup arthroplasty. Clin Orthop 1978;134:41–4.

[3] Wagner H. Surface replacement arthroplasty of the hip. Clin Orthop 1978;134:102–30.

[4] Howie DW, Campbell D, McGee M, et al. Wagner resurfacing hip arthroplasty. J Bone Joint Surg Am 1990;72:708–14.

[5] Amstutz HC, Graff-Radford A, Green T, et al. Tharies surface replacements. A review of the first 100 cases. Clin Orthop 1978;134:87–101.

[6] Amstutz HC, Sparling EA, Grigoris P, et al. Surface replacement: the hip replacement of the future? Hip Int 1998;8:187–207.

[7] Wagner M, Wagner H. Preliminary results of uncemented metal-on-metal stemmed and resurfacing hip replacement arthroplasty. Clin Orthop 1996;329S: S78–88.

[8] McMinn D, Treacy R, Lin K, et al. Metal-on-metal surface replacement of the hip: experience of the Mc Minn prosthesis. Clin Orthop 1996;329S:S89–98.

[9] De Smet KA, Pattyn C, et al. Early results of primary Birmingham Hip Resurfacing using a hybrid metal-on-metal couple. Hip Int 2002;12:158–62.

[10] McMinn DJW. Development of metal/metal hip resurfacing. Hip Int 2003;13:41–53.

[11] Amstutz HC, Beaulé PE, Dorey FJ, et al. Metal-on-metal hybrid surface arthroplasty: two to six-year follow-up study. J Bone Joint Surg Am 2004;86: 28–39.

[12] Beaulé P, Dorey F, Le Duff M, et al. Risk factors affecting early outcome of metal on metal surface arthroplasty of the hip in patients 40 years old and younger. Clin Orthop 2004;418:80–7.

[13] White SP, Beard DJ, Smith EJ. Resurfacing hip replacement—an audit of activity in the United Kingdom 2002–2003. Hip Int 2004;14:163–8.

[14] Chirodian N, Saw T, Villar R. Results of hybrid total hip replacement and resurfacing—Is there a difference? Hip Int 2004;14:169–73.

[15] Daniel J, Pynsent P, McMinn D. Metal-on-metal resurfacing of the hip in patients under the age of 55 years with osteoarthritis. J Bone Joint Surg Br 2004;86:177–84.

[16] Amstutz HC, Grigoris P. Metal-on-metal bearings in hip arthroplasty. Clin Orthop 1996;329S:S11–34.

[17] Chan FW, Bobyn D, Medley JB, et al. Wear and lubrication of metal-on-metal hip implants. Clin Orthop 1999;329:10–24.

[18] McKellop H, Park SH, Chiesa R, et al. In vivo wear of 3 types of metal-on-metal hip prostheses during 2 decades of use. Clin Orthop 1996;329S:S128–40.

[19] Charnley J. The long-term results of low-friction arthroplasty of the hip performed as a primary intervention. J Bone Joint Surg Br 1972;54:61–76.

[20] Engh CA, Massin P, et al. Roentgenographic assessment of the biologic fixation of porous-surfaced femoral components. Clin Orthop 1990;257:107–28.

[21] Epinette JA, Geesink RGT. Radiographic assessment of cementless hip prosthesis: ARA, a proposed new scoring system. Hydroxyapatite coated hip and knee arthroplasty. L'expansion Scientifique Française 1995; 51:114–26.

ELSEVIER
SAUNDERS

Orthop Clin N Am 36 (2005) 215–222

ORTHOPEDIC
CLINICS
OF NORTH AMERICA

Hydroxyapatite-Coated Femoral Implant in Metal-on-Metal Resurfacing Hip Arthroplasty: Minimum of Two Years Follow-Up

Anastasios K. Lilikakis, MD[a],*, Sarah L. Vowler, MSc[b],
Richard N. Villar, MS, FRCS[c]

[a]67 Pratinou Street, Athens 11634, Greece
[b]Centre for Applied Medical Statistics, Department of Public Health and Primary Care, Institute of Public Health,
University of Cambridge, Forvie Site, Robinson Way, Cambridge CB2 2SR, UK
[c]Cambridge Hip and Knee Unit, BUPA Cambridge Lea Hospital, 30 New Road, Impington, Cambridge CB4 9EL, UK

Mold hip arthroplasty was used in the earliest attempts to treat hip osteoarthritis [1], but the better results achieved with total hip replacement meant this latter technique soon gained favor with orthopaedic surgeons [2]. Surface arthroplasty reappeared in the 1970s, being developed simultaneously in different orthopaedic centers in Europe, Japan, and the United States, as a bone-preserving alternative to total hip replacement [3–9]. Initial encouraging results soon gave way to unacceptable failure rates, owing to acetabular loosening and femoral neck fractures [10–13]. These were attributed to the high wear rate of the thin polyethylene acetabular implant articulating with a large bearing surface [14–16]. Resurfacing once again was abandoned, although at the time it was noted that alternative bearings and biologic fixation could be the answer to the problems [16,17].

McMinn et al [18] and Wagner and Wagner [19] reintroduced resurfacing hip arthroplasty more than a decade ago, using a metal-on-metal articulation that has a low wear rate [20] and allows for a thinner acetabular implant and less bone resection in the ace-

tabulum. Hydroxyapatite was in use already and became the means of fixation of choice for the acetabular implant, but despite being tried successfully for the femoral implant, it was not adopted [18]. There are no studies reporting on the use of hydroxyapatite as a coating in the femoral side of hip resurfacing.

The authors report their preliminary experience with a minimum of 2 years of follow-up of hydroxyapatite coating as the means of fixation of the femoral head in hip resurfacing.

Between June 2001 and July 2002, the senior author performed 70 resurfacing arthroplasties in 66 patients. Twenty-nine were women (41.4%) and 37 were men (58.6%; 41 resurfacings). The mean age was 51.5 years (range, 23.3–72.7). The patients' mean height was 172 cm (range, 157–200; standard deviation [SD], 8.8). Their mean weight was 78 kg (range, 50–143; SD, 15.1). Mean body mass index was 26.3 (range, 19.8–37.2; SD, 3.8). The size of the femoral implants ranged from 40 mm (20 implants) to 52 mm (2 implants); the implant size used most frequently was 48 mm (31 implants). Seventeen implants were 44 mm. Twenty-six patients (37.1%) had a previous operation on the same hip, 20 of which were arthroscopies, 2 osteotomies with further removal of the implant, 1 biopsy of a femoral cyst, 1 open reduction of traumatic dislocation, 1 revascularization, and 1 open labrectomy. The preoperative

Dr. A. Lilikakis has received a research grant from Corin, Cirencester, United Kingdom, in support of this study.
* Corresponding author.
E-mail address: alilikakis@yahoo.com (A.K. Lilikakis).

diagnosis was osteonecrosis in 1 patient, chondrolysis in 1 patient, and osteoarthritis in the remaining 64 patients (68 hips).

The femoral and acetabular implants of the uncemented version of the Cormet 2000 (Corin; Cirencester, UK) were used throughout the study; they are made from high carbon cobalt chrome molybdenum alloy and are hot isostatic pressed and solution annealed (Fig. 1). In this design the heads are available in five sizes of 40–56 mm in 4-mm increments. There are two acetabular cups for each head size, 6 and 8 mm larger than the head, with a wall thickness of 3 and 4 mm, respectively. The cups are therefore available in 2-mm increments. The internal design of the resurfacing head includes three fins for rotational stability and a 1° taper on the cylindric section. The heads are fully coated in the inner surface with hydroxyapatite (HA) with the exception of the part of the stem outside the head, which is polished. The cup has four fins and features equatorial expansion such that a 50-mm cup is 25 mm in radius at the pole but 26 mm at the rim. The expansion is graduated from the pole to form a semi-elliptical profile and an over-reaming of 1 mm is advised for appropriate fixation. The acetabular component is coated with vacuum plasma sprayed titanium and hydroxyapatite. The bearing surfaces are polished to less than 0.05 microns Ra.

Interventions took place through a posterolateral approach and under general non-hypotensive anesthesia. The antithrombotic regime for all patients

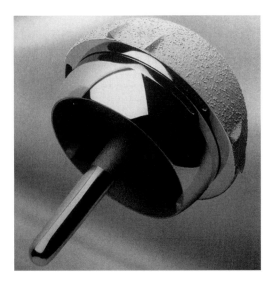

Fig. 1. The uncemented, hydroxyapatite-coated, metal-on-metal resurfacing arthroplasty Cormet (*From* Corin; Cirencester, UK; with permission.)

comprised 75 mg of aspirin for 30 days and the use of compressive stockings. Patients were mobilized the day after surgery, fully weightbearing in all but three cases for whom partial weightbearing for 2 weeks (one patient) and 6 weeks (two patients) was advised because of unsatisfying fixation of the acetabular component.

Patients were assessed preoperatively for pain and function with a modified Harris hip score (HHS) for which the maximum possible score was 91 points. Postoperatively they were mailed a questionnaire at 6 weeks, 6 months, and yearly thereafter. In addition to completing the HHS, they were asked to report on their satisfaction with the outcome of the procedure. Radiographs were obtained before and immediately after intervention, at 6 months and yearly thereafter, during regular follow-up with the aim of finding biomechanic parameters potentially associated with clinical evidence.

The following biomechanic parameters were evaluated on the anteroposterior preoperative radiographs of the pelvis centered on the pubis: the center of rotation of the hip, the femoral offset, and the neck-shaft angle. The hip center of rotation was localized with the use of the best-fit concentric circle [21]. The axis of the femoral shaft was realized by connecting two points in the middle of the intramedullary canal, one at 5 cm and one at 10 cm below the midpart of the lesser trochanter [22]. The axis of the femoral neck was determined by a line connecting the center of rotation with the middle of the neck isthmus [22]. The neck-shaft angle formed by these two axes was assessed preoperatively, whereas postoperatively the stem-shaft angle was measured. The difference of the postoperative minus the preoperative values constituted the varus or valgus displacement of the implant, with a positive difference reflecting a relative valgus position and a negative difference a relative varus position of the implant. The perpendicular distance (in centimeters) from the hip center of rotation to the femoral shaft axis was considered to be the femoral offset [21], and the difference between the preoperative and postoperative values constituted the change in offset. Preoperatively, patients commonly have an external rotation deformity that is eliminated postoperatively, showing a more varus stem-shaft angle, and in that respect the results of varus–valgus position and offset of the implant had limitations.

Anteroposterior displacement of the femoral stem was evaluated in the first lateral radiograph taken postoperatively, by calculating the angle between the stem and the neck axis. The neck axis connected the center of rotation of the cup and the middle of the neck isthmus. A stem was considered to be displaced when the angle was equal to or more than 10°, and neutral if less than 10° [23]. The presence of cysts in the femoral head and their size (smaller or larger than 1 cm) were recorded. In the first postoperative radiograph the presence of notching also was noted. Notching is a deficiency in the femoral neck cortex, most commonly laterally, created at reaming, usually caused by imprecise positioning of the guide wire.

Neck thinning has been observed previously in hip resurfacing [18,24]. To evaluate this, the authors measured the cup and the neck diameters at the cup-neck rim. To compensate for magnification in subsequent radiographs, the authors calculated the ratio of these two values, which were recorded after operation and at any available follow-up. A change of more than 10% in the cup-neck ratio (an absolute value of 0.1) was considered arbitrarily to be thinning of the neck.

The authors focused on the femoral component, because acetabular components of the same rationale are well studied and established [25]. Six patients did not respond to the questionnaires at the 2-year follow-up but were contacted by telephone. The radiographs of seven patients were not available for the study, limiting the total number of arthroplasties available for radiographic analysis to 63 (59 patients).

Statistical analysis was performed in SPSS 11.5 for Windows software (SPSS Inc; Chicago, IL). Kaplan-Meier estimates were used to calculate the survival rate of the implants. The Wilcoxon Signed Rank test was used for comparison for instances in which the data were not normally distributed, and the paired t test was used for instances in which the data were sufficiently normally distributed. Linear regression was used to investigate which factors effected the change in cup-neck ratio and any variable with a P value less than 0.1 univariately was included in a multivariate model.

Clinical results

The mean duration of follow-up was 28.5 months (range, 24.0–37.8 months). One acetabular component was revised because of aseptic loosening, and in one case both components were revised because of infection. Kaplan-Meier analysis demonstrated that the overall survival rate of the prosthesis was 97.1% (standard of error [SE], 0.02) and the mean survival time was 37.0 months (95% confidence interval [CI], 35.9–38.1), whereas the survival rate of the femoral component alone was 98.6% (SE, 0.014) and the mean survival time was 37.3 months (95% CI, 36.4–38.2). The mean HHS scores for pain and function preoperatively were 12.0 (range, 0–30) and 28.3 (range, 3–42), respectively, whereas postoperatively (at final follow-up) they were 39.3 (0–44) and 43.1 (9–47), respectively.

Analysis with the Wilcoxon Signed Rank test (Z) indicated that there was a significant improvement in pain and function at the final follow-up compared with preoperatively ($Z = -6.9$, $P < 0.0001$ for function; and $Z = -7.2$, $P < 0.0001$ for pain). At the final available follow-up, four patients were dissatisfied with the outcome of the procedure. One was the patient with deep infection before revision; two patients had pain (HHS of 20), whereas the other patient was the one with the displaced acetabular implant. The patient with the loose acetabular implant that was revised subsequently was satisfied after the revision.

Radiographic results

Of the 63 cases available for radiographic analysis, 39 hips (61.9%) had no cysts in the femoral head preoperatively, 16 hips (25.4%) had cysts smaller than 1 cm, and 8 hips (12.7%) had cysts greater than 1 cm. The mean neck-shaft angle was 130.1° (range, 114°–144°; SD, 6.3) and the mean offset preoperatively was 4.7 mm (range, 2.5–6.6; SD, 0.9). Postoperatively the stem-shaft angle was a mean of 140.8° (range, 124°–160°; SD, 7.0) and the offset was 4.7 mm (range, 2.6–6.8; SD, 0.9) (Figs. 2 and 3). Only one femoral implant was placed in varus ($-2°$) with the rest being in neutral or valgus, which represents the surgeon's intention to avoid varus placement of the implant. The mean change was 10.7° (range, $-2°$ varus to 24° valgus; SD, 6.8) and, with the use of the Wilcoxon Signed Rank test, this difference was statistically significant ($Z = -6.7$, $P < 0.0001$). The mean change in offset was -0.02 (range, -1.9–1.8; SD, 0.6), which, as analyzed with the t test, was not significant ($t = 0.2$; df = 64; $P = 0.8$).

Forty-seven (76.2%) of the 63 hips had no evidence of notching immediately after surgery. One hip (1.6%)—the varus placed cup—had inferomedial notching, and 15 hips (23.8%) had superolateral notching. The valgus placement in the hips with notching was a mean of 13.4°, whereas in those without notching it was 9.9° ($P = 0.08$). Fifty-three hips (84.1%) had a femoral cup in anteroposterior displacement of less than 10°, and in 10 hips (15.9%) displacement was 10° or more. There were no radiolucencies around the stem or any migration of the femoral implant in the series.

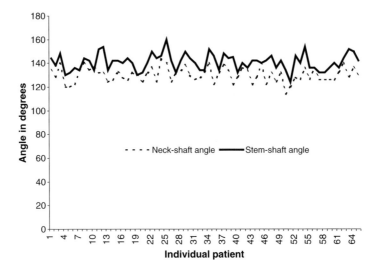

Fig. 2. Diagram of neck-shaft and stem-shaft angle values of individual patients.

The cup-neck ratio immediately after surgery was a mean of 1.05 (range, 1.0–1.3; SD, 0.06) indicating an oversize implant in some cases. The cup-neck ratio at last follow-up was 1.1 (range, 1.0–1.4; SD, 0.1) (Fig. 3). This difference was statistically significant as analyzed with the Wilcoxon Signed Rank test ($Z = -4.1$, $P < 0.0001$). In 26 hips the ratio did not change during follow-up, whereas in one hip an initial oversize had disappeared by the 6-month review. With a change in ratio of more than 10% defined as neck thinning, for 63 cases available for comparison, there was thinning in 17 (27%). In only one case did neck thinning occur in the superolateral cortex, whereas in all others it occurred in the inferomedial cortex (Fig. 4A–D). For cases in which there was a change in the cup-neck ratio, this was usually noticeable at 6 months as seen by post hoc analysis.

Regression analysis was used to distinguish the factors that affected significantly the change in cup-neck ratio. Demographic data (height, weight, age, gender, size of component used), clinical information (modified HHS, satisfaction), and radiographic parameters (neck-shaft angle, stem-shaft angle, change in angle, pre- and postoperative offset, change in off-

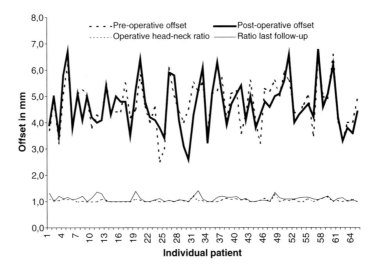

Fig. 3. Diagrams of pre- and postoperative offset values and the head–neck ratio immediately postoperatively and at last follow-up of individual patients.

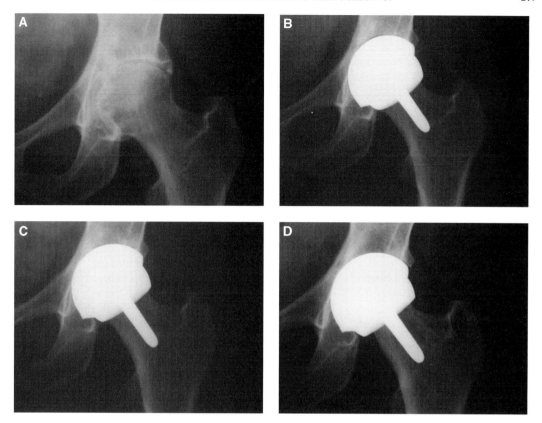

Fig. 4. (*A*) Preoperative radiograph of a 69-year-old woman with osteoarthritis. (*B*) Radiograph of the same patient 1 month after resurfacing arthroplasty. (*C*) Radiograph of the same patient at 6 months showing thinning already apparent at the inferomedial neck region. (*D*) Radiograph of the same patient 2 years after intervention showing further progression of neck thinning.

set, anteroposterior displacement of the cup, initial oversize of the implant, femoral cysts, notching) were included in the analysis.

Height, weight, and neck-shaft angle were included in the multivariate model, having passed the univariate screen. The height (standardized coefficient $\beta = 1.5$; $t = -2.3$; $P = 0.02$) significantly affected the change in cup-neck ratio, whereas weight did not reach statistical significance ($\beta = 2.1$; $t = 2$; $P = 0.06$). Height had a negative coefficient; taller patients seemed to be protected against neck thinning. Weight had a positive coefficient; heavier patients were more prone to neck thinning. This model, however, although based on the whole group, only explained 30% of the variance in change in cup-neck ratio, suggesting that other unidentified variables also influenced neck thinning.

There was no evidence of a correlation between the change in cup-neck ratio and the HHS for pain and function at final follow-up as calculated by the Spearman's rank correlation coefficient ($r_s = 0.1$ [95%

CI, $-0.2-0.3$]; $P = 1.0$ for function and $r_s = -0.1$ [95% CI, $-0.4-0.1$], $P = 0.4$ for pain). Height and weight were significantly correlated positively with the size of the femoral component ($r_s = 0.6$; 95% CI, $0.4-0.7$; $P < 0.001$ and $r_s = 0.6$; 95% CI, $0.4-0.7$; $P < 0.001$, respectively). The biomechanic measurements are summarized in Table 1.

Table 1

Mean values, ranges, and standard deviations of the biomechanical measurements

Radiographic variable	
Neck-shaft angle (degrees)	130.1 (114–144; SD, 6.26)
Stem-shaft angle (degrees)	140.8 (124–160; SD, 7.0)
Offset preoperatively (mm)	4.69 (2.5–6.6; SD, 0.86)
Offset postoperatively (mm)	4.64 (2.6–6.8; SD, 0.95)
Head–neck ratio postoperatively	1.05 (1.0–1.26; SD, 0.06)
Head–neck ratio at last follow-up	1.10 (1.0–1.4; SD, 0.10)

Complications

One hip was considered unstable intraoperatively and was treated with an abduction brace for 6 weeks. One patient sustained a pulmonary embolism 1 month after the procedure without further complications and one patient died 20 months after surgery for an unrelated reason. One patient developed a wound hematoma 10 days postoperatively and one patient developed a superficial wound infection; both were treated conservatively with no further problems. In one patient there was a 20° displacement of the cup within the first 6 months without further reoperation until final follow-up. One patient sustained a deep infection and was treated with a total hip replacement in another institution. Finally, one patient had aseptic loosening of the acetabular component, which was revised 15 months after the initial procedure with the next size up, whereas the femoral component was left in place. This patient was one of the three cases with unsatisfying initial fixation of the acetabular implant who were treated with partial weightbearing and who had low HHS for pain and function at the 6-week review. There were no dislocations in the series and only one patient had a grade II ectopic ossification as described by Brooker et al [26].

Resurfacing arthroplasty was reintroduced in the early 1990s and the short- to medium-term results have been promising [23,27]. Hydroxyapatite coating, inducing bone incorporation and thus enhancing fixation in orthopedic implants, was developed almost at the same time and has given good results [25]. It therefore seemed logical to incorporate hydroxyapatite as a coating to resurfacing arthroplasty. Although it has been adopted as a choice of fixation for the acetabulum by most manufacturers, it was not widely adopted for the femoral implant in resurfacing.

The authors' objective was to present the results of at least 2 years, experience with hydroxyapatite coating for the femoral implant in hip resurfacing. Only one femoral implant in this series of 70 cases was revised and this was because of infection. The 98.6% survival rate is promising and comparable with similar studies [23,27]. There were no cases of femoral loosening, neck fracture, or radiolucencies around the stem. Neck thinning has been a frequent radiologic finding, although it did not correlate with clinical symptoms.

Various factors have been implicated in femoral loosening and failure. Beaulé et al [24] recently have developed a surface arthroplasty risk index (SARI) indicating previous surgery, lighter weight, increased activity levels, and large femoral cysts as risk factors for early failure of cemented heads. Amstutz et al, from the same orthopedic center, have recently reported on 400 resurfacings with a minimum 2-year follow-up [23]. They also used the SARI and found that large cysts, height, female gender, and smaller component sizes in males are risk factors for femoral component loosening and stem radiolucencies. Varus placement of the femoral component [10,17,28] and notching of the neck [10,29,30] also have been implicated in femoral loosening and fracture of the neck. None of these risk factors has been shown to correlate with neck thinning in the authors' study. Increased height with reduced weight seemed to protect from thinning, which is in contrast with the Amstutz et al [23] and Beaulé et al [24] results. In their studies, height and reduced weight has been a risk factor for early failure. In the authors' series, neck thinning was not associated with failure, although it may predispose to femoral loosening in the future. The controversy also may represent the difference in biomechanic response between cemented and uncemented resurfaced heads, as the authors' model was able to interpret only 30% of the incidence of neck thinning.

Neck thinning has been reported in cemented resurfacing and has been considered to be an effect of remodeling with no clinical significance but one that may put the femoral neck at risk for fracture [18,24]. McMinn et al [18] have reported frequent neck thinning with no correlation with varus or valgus placement of the implant and no clinical implications. In a study by Beaulé et al [24], thinning was an infrequent finding that appeared in only two patients. In both studies, however, it was a superolateral thinning as opposed to the inferomedial one in the authors' series.

Possible causal factors of neck thinning are avascular necrosis caused by the femoral preparation at surgery and stress shielding owing to alteration of the biomechanic parameters of the hip [17]. Necrosis of the head after hip resurfacing has been a controversial issue [31], with most retrieval studies showing that the head remnant keeps a good blood supply [32,33].

De Waal and Huiskes [30] have published a biomechanic study on a two-dimensional finite element model of the TARA (Total Articular Resurfacing Arthroplasty, DePuy; Warsaw, IN) hip prosthesis with various stem lengths and different bonding distribution between implant and head. They showed that the distribution of bonding between implant and head influences stresses on the head and neck and that the presence of a stem contributes to load distribution by unloading the inferomedial cortex. This finding is in accordance with the three-dimensional finite element model of Watanabe et al [34], who found a stress concentration below the tip of the stem and also in the posteroinferior cup-rim, whereas stress shielding was present in the anterosuperior region of the neck.

These studies have been modeled on the cemented resurfacing arthroplasty, in which cement acts as filler and transmits forces to the neck. This is not true for HA-coated resurfacing. The authors believe that uncemented, HA-coated heads in resurfacing behave differently from cemented ones, and that in some cases the femoral neck may not be adequately loaded, with the stresses mainly distributed by the stem, causing stress shielding on the neck. Longer follow-up studies, biomechanic studies on an uncemented model, and retrieval analyses could appropriately explain if neck thinning is a harmless result of bone adaptation or a malignant phenomenon of bone resorption that jeopardizes the femoral neck.

Summary

The authors' preliminary results with a hydroxyapatite-coated femoral implant in metal-on-metal hip resurfacing have been promising with excellent survival rates and clinical outcomes. Longer follow-up studies are needed, particularly to interpret the clinical significance of neck thinning.

Acknowledgments

The authors wish to thank Clare Reinhardt, BSc, for her valuable contribution in the data provision for this study.

References

[1] Smith-Petersen MN. Evolution of mould arthroplasty of the hip joint. J Bone Joint Surg [Br] 1948;18B: 59–75.

[2] Charnley JC. Arthroplasty of the hip: a new operation. Lancet 1961;1:1129–32.

[3] Furuya K, Tsuchiya M, Kawachi S. Socket-cup arthroplasty. Clin Orthop 1978;134:41–4.

[4] Freeman MAR, Cameron HU, Brown GC. Cemented double cup arthroplasty of the hip: a 5-year experience with the ICLH prosthesis. Clin Orthop 1978;134: 45–52.

[5] Capello WN, Ireland PH, Trammel TR, Eicher P. Conservative total hip arthroplasty: a procedure to preserve bone stock. Clin Orthop 1978;134:59–74.

[6] Wagner H. Surface replacement arthroplasty of the hip. Clin Orthop 1978;134:102–30.

[7] Tanaka S. Surface replacement of the hip joint. Clin Orthop 1978;134:75–9.

[8] Trentani C, Vaccarino F. The Paltrinieri-Trentani hip joint resurface arthroplasty. Clin Orthop 1978;134: 36–40.

[9] Amstutz HC, Graff-Radford A, Gruen TA, Clarke IC. THARIES surface replacements: a review of the first 100 cases. Clin Orthop 1978;134:87–101.

[10] Jolley MN, Salvati EA, Brown GC. Early results and complications of surface replacement of the hip. J Bone Joint Surg [Am] 1982;64A:366–77.

[11] Head WC. Total articular resurfacing arthroplasty: analysis of component failure in sixty-seven hips. J Bone Joint Surg [Am] 1984;66A:28–34.

[12] Freeman MAR, Bradley GW. ICLH surface replacement of the hip: an analysis of the first 10 years. J Bone Joint Surg [Br] 1983;65B:405–11.

[13] Howie DW, Campbell D, McGee M, Cornish BL. Wagner resurfacing hip arthroplasty: the results of one hundred consecutive arthroplasties after eight to ten years. J Bone Joint Surg [Am] 1990;72A: 708–13.

[14] Howie DW, Cornish BL, Vernon-Roberts B. Resurfacing hip arthroplasty: classification of loosening and the role of prosthesis wear particles. Clin Orthop Rel Res 1990;255:144–59.

[15] Mai MT, Schmalzried TP, Dorey FJ, Campbell PA, Amstutz HC. The contribution of frictional torque to loosening at the cement-bone interface in Tharies hip replacement. J Bone Joint Surg [Am] 1996;78A: 505–11.

[16] Black J, Sholtes V. Biomaterial aspects of surface replacement arthroplasty of the hip. Symposium on Surface Arthroplasty of the Hip. Orthop Clin N Am 1982;13(4):709–28.

[17] Clarke IC. Biomechanics. Symposium on Surface Arthroplasty of the Hip. Orthop Clin N Am 1982; 13(4):681–707.

[18] McMinn D, Treacy R, Lin K, Pynsent P. Metal on metal surface replacement of the hip: experience of the McMinn prosthesis. Clin Orthop Rel Res 1996; 329(Suppl):S89–98.

[19] Wagner M, Wagner H. Preliminary results of uncemented metal on metal stemmed and resurfacing hip replacement arthroplasty. Clin Orthop Rel Res 1996; 329(Suppl):S78–88.

[20] Anissian HL, Stark A, Gustafson A, Good V, Clarke IC. Metal-on-metal bearing in hip prostheses generates 100-fold less wear debris than metal-on-polyethylene. Acta Orthop Scand 1999;70:578–82.

[21] Silva M, Lee KH, Heisel C, Dela Rosa MA, Schmalzried TP. The biomechanical results of total hip resurfacing arthroplasty. J Bone Joint Surg [Am] 2004;86A:40–6.

[22] Grecula MJ, Thomas JA, Kreuzer SW. Impact of implant design on femoral head hemiresurfacing arthroplasty. Clin Orthop 2004;418:41–7.

[23] Amstutz HA, Beaulé PE, Dorey FJ, Le Duff MJ, Campbell PA, Gruen TA. Metal-on-metal hybrid surface arthroplasty: two- to six-year follow-up study. J Bone Joint Surg [Am] 2004;86A:28–39.

[24] Beaulé PE, Dorey FJ, LeDuff M, Gruen T, Amstutz HC. Risk factors affecting outcome of metal-on-metal surface arthroplasty of the hip. Clin Orthop 2004;418: 87–93.

[25] Epinette JA, Manley MT, Duthoit E. Long-term results with the HA-coated Arc2F in primary hip surgery. In: Epinette JA, Manley MT, editors. Fifteen years of clinical experience with hydroxyapatite coatings in joint arthroplasty. France: Springer-Verlag; 2004. p. 313–24.

[26] Brooker AF, Bowerman JW, Robinson RA, Riley LH. Ectopic ossification following total hip replacements. Incidence and a method of classification. J Bone Joint Surg [Am] 1973;55A:1629–32.

[27] Daniel J, Pynsent PB, McMinn DJW. Metal-on-metal resurfacing of the hip in patients under the age of 55 years with osteoarthritis. J Bone Joint Surg [Br] 2004;86B:177–84.

[28] Freeman MAR. Some anatomical and mechanical considerations relevant to the surface replacement of the femoral head. Clin Orthop 1978;134:19–24.

[29] Markolf KL, Amstutz HA. Mechanical strength of the femur following resurfacing and conventional total hip replacement. Clin Orthop Rel Res 1980;147: 170–80.

[30] De Waal Malefijt MC, Huiskes R. A clinical, radiological and biomechanical study of the TARA hip prosthesis. Arch Orthop Trauma Surg 1993;112:220–5.

[31] Bogoch ER, Fornasier VL, Capello WN. The femoral head remnant in resurfacing arthroplasty. Clin Orthop Rel Res 1982;167:92–105.

[32] Campbell P, Mirra J, Amstutz HC. Viability of femoral heads treated with resurfacing arthroplasty. J Arthroplasty 2000;15:120–2.

[33] Howie DW, Cornish BL, Vernon-Roberts B. The viability of the femoral head after resurfacing hip arthroplasty in humans. Clin Orthop Rel Res 1993;291: 171–84.

[34] Watanabe Y, Shiba N, Matsuo S, Higuchi F, Tagawa Y, Inoue A. Biomechanical study of the resurfacing hip arthroplasty: finite element analysis of the femoral component. J Arthroplasty 2000;15:505–11.

ELSEVIER
SAUNDERS

Orthop Clin N Am 36 (2005) 223 – 230

ORTHOPEDIC
CLINICS
OF NORTH AMERICA

Surface Arthroplasty in Young Patients with Hip Arthritis Secondary to Childhood Disorders

Harlan C. Amstutz, MD[a],*, Edwin P. Su, MD[b], Michel J. Le Duff, MA[a]

[a]Joint Replacement Institute, Orthopaedic Hospital, 2400 South Flower Street, Los Angeles, CA 90007, USA
[b]Hospital for Special Surgery, 535 East 70th Street, New York, NY 10021, USA

Legg-Calvé-Perthes disease (LCP) and slipped capital femoral epiphysis (SCFE) are disorders of the hip that occur in children and adolescents, which may result in degenerative joint disease in adulthood. Although these processes are self-limited, LCP and SCFE often cause alterations in proximal femoral anatomy that affect joint mechanics, create impingement, and lead to the development of degenerative joint disease [1–3]. Frequently, this secondary osteoarthritis occurs in the third or fourth decade of life as a consequence of these childhood conditions [4,5].

Treatment of end-stage osteoarthritis is especially challenging in these patients because of their young age, the aberrant proximal femoral geometry, previous surgery often with retained hardware, leg length discrepancy, and a relative acetabular dysplasia or retroversion, which adds to early joint damage. LCP often results in a broad, flattened head (coxa plana) and a short, wide, anteverted femoral neck (Fig. 1); the residual deformity of SCFE often is a "pistol-grip" deformity with a retroverted head on a wide femoral neck (Fig. 2) [6].

Surface arthroplasty of the hip is emerging as a treatment option for younger patients with end-stage coxarthrosis because of its bone-conserving nature, joint stability, and the ability to easily convert to a total hip replacement should there be a femoral failure [7]. Hip resurfacing requires downsizing the femoral head diameter to the margins of the femoral neck,

especially when the neck is wide and full leg equalization may not be possible. Normal biomechanics and leg length discrepancy may be more simply corrected with a conventional total hip replacement, but the problems of proximal stress shielding and revision of stem-type devices remain.

The low head-to-neck ratio, short neck length, and abnormal position of the head relative to the neck make it a challenge to resurface without violating the integrity of the neck, to increase leg length, and to orient the components to avoid impingement. O'Hara [8] recently reported on a series of patients in which a concurrent osteotomy, trochanteric osteotomy with advancement, or both were performed as a one- or two-stage procedure in an attempt to normalize the anatomy before undertaking resurfacing. Occasionally, it may be necessary to notch the femoral neck to resurface without removing excessive acetabular bone.

The purposes of this study were to quantitatively describe the proximal femoral anatomy (specifically, the head-neck relationship) and to evaluate the safety and efficacy of surface arthroplasty for these technically challenging patients with altered proximal femoral geometry due to LCP and SCFE.

Materials and methods

Patient cohort

The authors performed a retrospective review of all patients with arthritis of the hip secondary to LCP or SCFE who underwent surface arthroplasty between 1996 and 2002 at the Joint Replacement In-

This work was supported by the Los Angeles Orthopaedic Hospital Foundation.
* Corresponding author.
E-mail address: hamstutz@laoh.ucla.edu (H.C. Amstutz).

orthopedic.theclinics.com

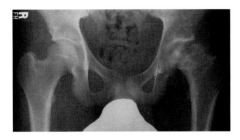

Fig. 1. Anteroposterior radiograph of an 18-year-old man with grade 3 osteoarthritis [14–16] of the left hip secondary to LCP. Note the flattened femoral head on a short, wide femoral neck. There is a congruent nonspherical shape to the articular surfaces with large femoral cysts. The patient exhibited 30° of combined ab-adduction, 25° of rotation, and 100° of flexion.

Table 1
Summary of patient demographic information (n = 25)

Parameter	Mean	SD	Range	n (%)
Age at surgery (y)	38.1	11.8	15–57	—
Weight (kg)	89.2	21.1	59–136	—
Height (cm)	177	7.9	161–193	—
Body mass index	28.5	6.7	18.4–43.4	—
Male	—	—	—	19 (90%)
Female	—	—	—	2 (10%)
Charnley class A	—	—	—	12 (57%)
Charnley class B	—	—	—	10 (43%)
Charnley class C	—	—	—	0 (0%)

stitute. The senior author (H.C.A.) performed all of the operations in a consecutive series of 522 resurfacings. Twenty-one patients with end-stage hip arthritis secondary to LCP or SCFE underwent 25 surface arthroplasties in this study period.

Eleven patients (14 hips) with LCP and 10 patients (11 hips) with SCFE underwent surface replacement. The average age at the time of surgery was 38.1 years (range, 18.2–57.9 years). Twenty patients were men, 3 of whom had bilateral surface arthroplasties; only 2 patients in the SCFE cohort were women. Nine hips (all with SCFE) had undergone 10 previous operations (8 femoral head pinnings and 2 femoral osteotomies). The patient demographics are summarized in Table 1.

The implant

The surface arthroplasties were done as part of the United States Food and Drug Administration multi-

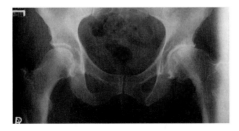

Fig. 2. Anteroposterior radiograph of a 41-year-old man with grade 3 osteoarthritis [14–16] of the left hip secondary to SCFE. Note the relationship of the head to the neck, with a characteristic "pistol-grip" deformity and evidence of the previous pinning. There is extensive cystic degeneration inferiorly. The patient had a 20° external rotation contracture.

center investigational device exemption (IDE) study utilizing the Conserve Plus prosthesis (Wright Medical Technologies, Arlington, Tennessee) between the years 1996 to 2000 and as part of the "IDE continued access" granted for this device by the Food and Drug Administration between the years 2000 and 2002. The components used, the surgical technique, and the postoperative management were previously described by Amstutz et al [9]. All of the sockets had the standard 5-mm wall thickness. The first LCP hip arthroplasty was performed with a trochanteric osteotomy; the rest of the series with a posterior approach. Intraoperative photographs of the prepared femoral head were taken to record the bony defects and remaining support for the femoral component after bone preparation prior to implantation. All of the earliest cases were performed without cementation of the metaphyseal stem but after April 2000, the stem was cemented in when the cystic defects were greater than 1 cm.

Three hips with an etiology of SCFE, all previously pinned, were paste grafted after femoral head preparation to fill up pin tracts and large cystic defects. The most recent grafted case also had the stem cemented in. Four hips (all SCFE) had pre-existing hardware in situ at the time of surgery. The hardware was removed in three cases and left in place in one case because it could not be removed.

Radiographic follow-up

Standardized pre- and postoperative anteroposterior pelvis and cross-table (Johnson) lateral radiographs were evaluated for each patient by an independent reviewer (E.P.S.)—an orthopedic surgeon specialized in adult reconstruction and joint arthroplasty at the Hospital for Special Surgery. Radiolucencies around the acetabular cup were reported according to the DeLee and Charnley classification [10], and radiolucencies around the femoral metaphyseal stem were recorded as described by Amstutz et al [7]. Radiographic parameters concerning the head and neck relationship were measured pre- and postoperatively. These parameters included head-to-neck ratio, anterior head offset ratio, posterior head offset ratio, and lateral head offset ratio.

Concentric circles that best fit the contour of the femoral heads were used to reconstruct a sphere and allow the measurement of head diameter. The head-to-neck ratio was calculated by dividing the head diameter by the width of the femoral neck at its midpoint. The anterior head offset ratio was measured as described by Eijer et al [11] and represents the ratio of the distance between the anterior cortex of the neck and the anterior apex of the head over the diameter of the head, with all measurements made perpendicularly to the longitudinal axis of the neck on the lateral radiograph (Fig. 3). The posterior head offset ratio was measured in a similar fashion on the lateral radiograph, as was the lateral head offset ratio on the anteroposterior radiograph. Postoperative radiographs were also analyzed for component position as described previously by Amstutz et al [7]. In addition, an attempt was made to evaluate the level of con-

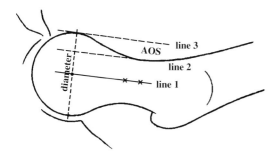

Fig. 3. On the lateral radiograph, the anterior head-neck offset was determined as follows: a line was drawn through the axis of the neck (thus not necessarily through the center of the head) (*line 1*). Another line was drawn parallel to the first one along the anterior cortex of the neck (in the axial radiograph, this is the upper side) (*line 2*). Another line was drawn parallel to the first one along the anterior outer part of the head (*line 3*). The offset was determined as the distance between lines 2 and 3. The diameter of the head was determined 90° to the three lines through the center of the head. The offset ratio was calculated by dividing the head-neck offset by the diameter of the head. (*From* Eijer H, Leunig M, Mahomed M, et al. Cross-table lateral radiographs for screening of anterior femoral head-neck offset in patients with femoro-acetabular impingement. Hip Int 2001; 11:37–41; with permission.)

gruity of the joint from the anteroposterior radiographs using the following criteria:

0 = Congruity—fairly spherical head and constant joint space

1 = Mild incongruity—head out of round but follows the acetabular contour

2 = Moderate incongruity—flattened head only allows motion in sagittal plane

3 = Severe incongruity—inversion of head curvature and large joint space discrepancies

Of the 25 hips in the study population, 23 had complete pre- and postoperative radiographs available for review.

Clinical follow-up

The patients were followed postoperatively at 6 weeks, 6 months, 1 year, and yearly thereafter. Hip range of motion (ROM), SF-12, and University of California Los Angeles (UCLA) hip scores were recorded pre- and postoperatively. Twenty-three hips in the study population had complete clinical follow-up data obtained by the senior investigator (H.C.A.). Two LCP patients were lost to follow-up after 13 months.

Statistical analysis

Comparisons were carried out within the study cohort (paired Student t test) between pre- and postoperative scores and between the study cohort (homoscedastic Student t test) and the rest of the patients implanted during the same period with the same prosthesis but with etiologies other than LCP or SCFE (n = 497). All comparisons of outcome measures were performed using Microsoft Excel 2002 (Redmond, Washington). P values less than 0.05 were deemed statistically significant.

Results

Clinical results

The average duration of clinical follow-up was 4.7 years (range, 2.7–8.1 years). Bilateral femoral components in a patient with LCP demonstrated radiographic evidence of migration and required bilateral conversion to total hip arthroplasty at 55 months post surgery. In the remainder of the study patients, the preoperative UCLA pain, walking, function, and activity scores improved significantly in

Table 2
Summary of the University of California Los Angeles and
SF-12 scores

Rating system	Score		
	Preoperative mean (range)	Latest follow-up mean (range)	P
Legg-Calvé-Perthes disease cohort (n = 12)			
UCLA hip score			
Pain	2.9 (1–5)	9.5 (8–10)	<0.0001
Walking	6.6 (5–8)	9.3 (8–10)	<0.0001
Function	6.1 (3–10)	9.2 (8–10)	<0.0001
Activity	4.9 (2–8)	7.7 (6 to 10)	<0.0001
SF-12			
Physical	32.7 (23.0–48.7)	52.9 (31.3–62.1)	<0.0001
Mental	47.0 (20.9–64.4)	42.9 (10.5–60.7)	NS
Slipped capital femoral epiphysis cohort (n=11)			
UCLA hip score			
Pain	2.9 (1–5)	8.9 (8–10)	<0.0001
Walking	4.7 (3–9)	9.9 (9–10)	<0.0001
Function	4.9 (4–9)	9.7 (8–10)	<0.0001
Activity	4.1 (4–6)	7.3 (6–9)	<0.0001
SF-12			
Physical	28.8 (21.1–35.5)	53.9 (40.7–58.2)	<0.0001
Mental	38.2 (14.0–58.3)	49.9 (24.4–57.6)	NS

both groups. At an average follow-up of 5 months (range, 2–15), nine patients (nine hips) reported minor activity-related pain. The pain location was distributed as follows: front/groin (one hip), back/buttocks (one hip), side (one hip), and any combination of the above (six hips). Postoperative SF-12 physical component scores also improved significantly in both cohorts, whereas mental component scores did not change significantly.

The UCLA and SF-12 scores are summarized in Table 2.

Compared with the cohort of patients who underwent resurfacing for other reasons during this time

period, the LCP and SCFE study group had a significantly lower preoperative pain score (2.9 versus 3.5, $P < 0.02$). Postoperatively, the SF-12 physical score of the study group was not significantly different from the larger cohort. Interestingly, the postoperative SF-12 mental score was significantly lower (46.1 versus 53.8, $P < 0.001$); however, two patients (four hips) from the series suffered from long-standing depression that was pre-existing at the time of surgery. When these patients' scores were removed, there was no difference in SF-12 mental component scores between the series and the rest of the cohort (52.79 versus 53.8, $P = 0.65$).

Preoperatively, the LCP cohort averaged 76° of flexion arc, 4° of internal rotation, and 15° of external rotation. The SCFE cohort had 67° of flexion arc, −17° of internal rotation, and 24° of external rotation preoperatively. After surface arthroplasty, the amount of flexion, internal rotation, and external rotation increased significantly in the LCP and SCFE group. The amount of flexion contracture decreased significantly in both groups of patients. The preoperative and postoperative ranges of motion are summarized in Table 3.

In comparing the hip ROM in the study population to the larger cohort who had surface arthroplasty for other reasons, preoperative flexion was found to be significantly less (93.4° versus 103.7°, $P < 0.003$), with a greater preoperative flexion contracture (22.4° versus 16.3°, $P < 0.04$). The postoperative flexion was also less in the study population (115.8° versus 125.1°, $P < 0.003$), but the net gain in flexion arc was comparable (36.7° versus 36.4°, $P = 0.94$).

Limb length discrepancies were present in 11 patients preoperatively. The discrepancy was <1 cm in 6 patients, 1 to 2 cm in 3 patients, and 2 to 3 cm in 2 patients. Of these 11 patients, the limb lengths were

Table 3
Summary of hip range of motion

Motion	Degrees		
	Preoperative mean (range)	Latest follow-up mean (range)	P
Legg-Calvé-Perthes disease cohort			
Flexion	98.5 (70–130)	117.5 (110–135)	<0.0001
Flexion contracture	23.1 (0–50)	1.3 (0–5)	<0.02
Internal rotation	4.2 (−10–20)	30.7 (15–60)	<0.0001
External rotation	14.6 (0–30)	33.6 (25–40)	<0.02
Slipped capital femoral epiphysis cohort			
Flexion	87.3 (75–110)	118 (105–130)	<0.0001
Flexion contracture	20 (0–45)	5.2 (0–25)	<0.02
Internal rotation	−16.8 (−45–10)	35 (20–50)	<0.0001
External rotation	24.1 (0–45)	40.5 (20–55)	<0.001

postoperatively equalized in 6 patients, 3 were maintained with the same amount of discrepancy, and 2 decreased their discrepancy by at least 1 cm.

Postoperative Trendelenburg sign was negative for all but four hips that exhibited a level sign, in addition to the two hips (one patient) that were revised for femoral loosening and showed a positive sign at the time of revision. Surprisingly, none of the patients showed any obvious gait disturbances at the last follow-up.

Preoperative radiographic analysis

The head-to-neck ratio was 1.27 (range, 1.07–1.53) in the LCP group and 1.28 (range, 1.17–1.42) in the SCFE group. For comparison, the authors also measured the femoral neck width of the contralateral, healthy hip in Charnley class A patients (n = 12) and found it significantly lower than the neck width on the operated hip (34.2 versus 42.0, respectively, after

correction for 20% magnification, $P = 0.0002$). The anterior, posterior, and lateral offset ratios were 0.18, 0.25, and 0.11, respectively, in the LCP group; in the SCFE group, they were 0.20, 0.25, and 0.12, respectively (Table 4). Neck-shaft angles were 131° on the anteroposterior radiograph and 30° on the lateral radiograph in the LCP cohort; angles were 138° and 25°, respectively, in the SCFE cohort.

The congruity of the joint on anteroposterior radiograph was correlated to the size of cysts recorded at the time of surgery ($r = 0.47$, $P < 0.05$). The average acetabular index was 44° (range, 41°–50°) in the LCP cohort and 41° (range, 34°–48°) in the SCFE group.

Intraoperative

All 25 hips in this study cohort had successful implantation of a surface arthroplasty at the time of surgery; that is, in no cases did the distorted proximal

Table 4
Summary of preoperative radiographic parameters

Hip #	Gender	Head/neck ratio	Anterior offset ratio	Lateral offset ratio	Posterior offset ratio
Legg-Calve-Perthes disease cohort					
30	M	1.53	0.20	0.10	0.18
206	M	1.07	0.18	0.18	0.33
207	M	1.26	0.23	0.10	0.31
248	M	1.46	0.22	0.16	0.31
249	M	1.39	0.16	0.07	0.18
310	M	1.26	0.21	0.15	0.18
375	M	1.44	0.10	0.12	0.18
381	M	1.23	0.27	0.12	0.35
385	M	1.09	0.16	0.00	0.38
388	M	1.39	0.24	0.04	0.28
403	M	1.21	0.15	0.19	0.02
410	M	1.21	0.18	0.14	0.33
437	M	1.18	0.27	0.21	0.29
516	M	1.11	0.18	0.18	0.22
Averages		**1.27**	**0.20**	**0.13**	**0.25**
Slipped capital femoral epiphysis cohort					
4	F	1.30	—	0.15	—
138	M	1.40	0.24	0.10	0.43
160	M	1.20	0.20	0.06	0.20
169	M	1.23	0.14	0.10	0.18
172	M	1.16	0.19	0.15	0.29
325	M	1.41	0.27	0.21	0.23
331	M	1.42	0.22	0.16	0.25
420	F	1.17	0.20	0.16	0.26
456	M	1.22	0.20	0.09	0.41
521	M	1.25	0.20	0.06	0.28
522	M	1.25	0.16	0.10	0.15
Averages		**1.27**	**0.20**	**0.12**	**0.27**

Abbreviations: F, female; M, male.

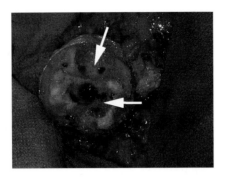

Fig. 4. Intraoperative photograph of the case shown in Fig. 1 (patient with osteoarthritis secondary to LCP) demonstrating the extensive femoral cystic degeneration. Arrows show the curetted cystic defects after completion of the femoral head preparation.

femoral anatomy preclude surface arthroplasty. In 10 cases, the proximal femoral anatomy was altered. A medial notch was made partially through the thick cortex in 4 hips to prepare the femoral head for the maximum femoral component size available then (1 case) or to avoid removing too much acetabular bone where the acetabular walls were thin (3 cases). ROM was optimized by carefully removing bone from the anterior acetabular wall and osteophytes from the femoral neck in 4 cases. In 3 cases, an ostectomy of the posterior intertrochanteric ridge (approximately $1.5 \times 1.5 \times 2.5-3$ cm) was performed to remove impingement in external rotation.

Large femoral cysts (>1 cm) were noted at the time of femoral preparation in 18 hips (Fig. 4), five cysts were larger than 2 cm (three of which were bone grafted). Compared to the rest of the series, this subgroup presented greater cystic degeneration ($P = 0.019$).

The average size of the femoral component was 48.5 mm (range, 44–52 mm) and the corresponding acetabular component was 10 mm larger. Femoral stems were cemented in 8 of the 14 hips in the LCP group and 2 of the 11 hips in the SCFE group.

Postoperative radiographic analysis

The mean duration of radiographic follow-up was 32.1 months (range, 3–96 months). The stem shaft angle averaged 140.3° in the anteroposterior plane and averaged 6.3° of posterior-to-anterior orientation compared with the main axis of the neck on the lateral plane. Two hips in the SCFE group demonstrated penetration of the anterior neck with the femoral stem. Two additional hips in the SCFE and one hip in the LCP group had contact of the stem with the anterior femoral neck.

Postoperative head offsets and head-to-neck ratios did not change significantly in either group of patients.

In the LCP cohort, one patient with bilateral resurfacings had radiolucencies about the femoral stem in zones 1 and 2 on the left side and demonstrated stem migration on the right side. This patient underwent conversion to bilateral total hip arthroplasty at 55 months post surgery. No patients had evidence of acetabular component migration, three patients had lucencies in zone III, and one patient had incomplete radiolucencies in two zones of the acetabulum. In the SCFE group, there were no radiolucencies about the femoral stem and there was one incomplete acetabular lucency in two zones.

Complications

One patient in the LCP cohort required bilateral conversions to total hip arthroplasty with a unipolar ball and Anthropometric Total Hip uncemented stem (Kinamed, Camarillo, California) at 55 months post surgery due to progressive femoral component migration. No other reoperations were performed on this study cohort. No hip dislocations or femoral neck fractures occurred in either group. One patient had a transient postoperative femoral nerve palsy that resolved.

Discussion

Surface arthroplasty has been advocated as a treatment for hip arthritis in younger patients because of its bone-conserving nature, joint stability, and the ability to easily convert to a total hip replacement should there be a femoral failure. It is a technically difficult operation to perform in patients with normal proximal femoral anatomy because of the need to maintain femoral neck integrity [9,12]. In patients who have aberrant proximal femoral geometry due to LCP or SCFE, this procedure is even more demanding.

In the LCP group, the head was often enlarged and flattened, resulting in a shorter femoral neck and head length. The shorter length of the femoral neck and head, along with the loss of height, made it difficult to restore limb length and the biomechanics of the hip and to prepare the bone to allow proper seating of the femoral component without damaging the neck. With the SCFE patients, the head was offset medially and posteriorly. The preoperative anterior offset ratio averaged 0.20. In a previous study, Eijer et al [11] found that asymptomatic hips had an anterior offset of 0.21 and symptomatic hips had an offset of 1.3. The authors' results do not seem to confirm anterior femoroacetabular impingement as a major contributing factor to the development of arthritis. The authors also looked at the lateral offset ratio, which averaged only 0.12 in the whole group, possibly indicating a tilting of the head medially. A search of the literature revealed no point of comparison for this number, but the authors found it useful in characterizing the relationship of the head to the neck.

Despite these anatomic abnormalities, surface arthroplasty was successfully performed in all of the study patients. Of the 25 hip resurfacings that were performed, 23 have survived (92%) at an average of 4.7 years. One bilateral resurfacing was converted to total hip arthroplasty at 55 months post surgery because of femoral component loosening. In reviewing this patient's data, factors contributing to femoral loosening included a relatively small head size (46 mm), presence of large femoral cysts, a high activity level (10 on the UCLA scale), and a surface arthroplasty risk index of 5 on each hip [13]. His resurfacing was performed prior to the senior author's (H.C.A.) modification of the technique to cement the stem in high-risk cases. Since instituting this technique modification in 2000, 8 of 9 hips with LCP and 2 hips with SCFE have had the stem inserted with cement, and none of these hips have shown any signs of radiographic loosening. The authors did not find any relationship between preoperative radiographic parameters and outcomes. At the latest follow-up period, the lack of evidence of loosening in the other patients is encouraging despite the presence of large cysts. Nevertheless, the correlation of cystic degeneration to incongruity should lead to careful follow-up of these patients so that surgery might be considered prior to severe cystic degeneration, which could ultimately affect durability.

Surface arthroplasty significantly improved UCLA hip scores, SF-12 physical scores, and ROM in all patients. Limb length discrepancy was diminished in all patients. There were no dislocations or femoral neck fractures. Radiographs revealed three hips in which the femoral component stem abutted and two SCFE hips in which the stem penetrated the anterior femoral cortex. This positioning of the femoral component was most likely caused by difficulty in visualizing the head-to-neck relationship in two of the authors' earliest cases (body mass index of 42 and 35), inadvertently directing the stem along the contours of the head rather than the neck. Despite these findings, the patients were asymptomatic and maintained high UCLA hip scores at 5.5 and 8 years post surgery, with modest activity levels of 6 and 7.

Although hip resurfacing is a technically difficult operation in these patients because of a flattened head and short neck in LCP and a wide femoral neck with retroverted heads in SCFE, the results to date have been encouraging. Despite the inability to fully correct the abnormal anatomic and biomechanical parameters and leg length discrepancy, all of the patients were pleased with the normalization of their hips, presumably due in part to their prior long-standing disability. Although all patients had a functional ROM, the lack of full restitution of ROM could be due to the preoperative presence of very stiff hips, impingement due to the short neck, or both. The postoperative initial recovery was not different from resurfaced hips that had other etiologies; however, obtaining maximum ROM and strength took longer. By taking extra care to avoid notching the neck on the anterior and lateral tension sides, satisfactory results can be achieved with a low incidence of complications. The use of thinner acetabular components (3.5-mm wall thickness) in addition to femoral sizes up to 56 mm should allow a better postoperative restoration of the head-to-neck and offset ratios and avoid the need for neck notching. Should notching be necessary, however, the authors recommend doing it medially where the cortex is thicker, rather than laterally.

References

[1] Catterall A. Legg-Calve-Perthes syndrome. Clin Orthop 1981;158:41–52.
[2] Leunig M, Casillas MM, Hamlet M, et al. Slipped capital femoral epiphysis: early mechanical damage to the acetabular cartilage by a prominent femoral metaphysis. Acta Orthop Scand 2000;71:370–5.
[3] Stulberg SD, Cooperman DR, Wallensten R. The natural history of Legg-Calve-Perthes disease. J Bone Joint Surg Am 1981;63:1095–108.
[4] Weinstein S. Legg-Calve-Perthes disease: results of long-term follow-up. Hip 1985;28–37.
[5] McAndrew MP, Weinstein SL. A long-term follow-up of Legg-Calve-Perthes disease. J Bone Joint Surg Am 1984;66:860–9.
[6] Goodman DA, Feighan JE, Smith AD, et al. Sub-clinical slipped capital femoral epiphysis. Relationship to osteoarthrosis of the hip. J Bone Joint Surg Am 1997;79:1489–97.
[7] Amstutz HC, Beaule PE, Dorey FJ, et al. Metal-on-metal hybrid surface arthroplasty: two to six-year follow-up study. J Bone Joint Surg Am 2004;86:28–39.
[8] O'Hara J. Hip resurfacing and femoral osteotomy in the treatment of complex hip deformity. Presented at the Combined Orthopaedic Associations. Sydney, Australia, October 24–29, 2004.

[9] Amstutz HC, Beaule PE, Le Duff MJ. Hybrid metal on metal surface arthroplasty of the hip. Op Tech Orthop 2001;11:253–62.

[10] DeLee JG, Charnley J. Radiological demarcation of cemented sockets in total hip replacement. Clin Orthop 1976;121:20–32.

[11] Eijer H, Leunig M, Mahomed M, et al. Cross-table lateral radiographs for screening of anterior femoral head-neck offset in patients with femoro-acetabular impingement. Hip Int 2001;11:37–41.

[12] Amstutz HC, Grigoris P, Dorey FJ. Evolution and future of surface replacement of the hip. J Orthop Sci 1998;3:169–86.

[13] Beaule PE, Dorey FJ, LeDuff M, et al. Risk factors affecting outcome of metal-on-metal surface arthroplasty of the hip. Clin Orthop 2004;418:87–93.

[14] Tonnis D, Heinecke A. Acetabular and femoral anteversion: relationship with osteoarthritis of the hip. J Bone Joint Surg Am 1999;81:1747–70.

[15] Bruckl R, Hepp W, Tonnis D. Eine abgrenzung normaler und dysplastischer hüftgelenke durch den hüftwert. Arch Orthop Trauma Surg 1972;74:13–32.

[16] Busse J, Gasteiger W, Tonnis D. Eine neue methode zur röntgenologischen beurteilung eines hüftgelenkesder hüftwert. Arch Orthop Trauma Surg 1972;72:1–9.

ELSEVIER
SAUNDERS

Orthop Clin N Am 36 (2005) 231–242

ORTHOPEDIC
CLINICS
OF NORTH AMERICA

Resurfacing Arthroplasty in Osteonecrosis of the Hip

Michael J. Grecula, MD

*Department of Orthopaedics and Rehabilitation, University of Texas Medical Branch, 301 University Boulevard, Route 0476,
Galveston, TX 77555, USA*

The ideal treatment for osteonecrosis of the femoral head would preserve the femoral head, provide complete relief of pain, have minimal morbidity, and would allow the patient to resume full activity without restrictions. Bone-preserving treatments are successful when treating early stages of osteonecrosis, but these results decline when used to treat more-advanced stages of the disease. Because femoral head osteonecrosis is a progressive disease in most cases, it is recommended to treat the disease at the earliest possible stage. Observation with protected weight bearing has shown poor results, with only a 22% survival rate at a mean follow-up of 34 months [1]. Pharmacologic treatments, electrical stimulation, high-energy shock-wave therapy, ultrasonography, and hyperbaric oxygen therapy are all considered experimental at the present time [2]. Core decompression has markedly variable success dependent on the size, stage, and underlying cause of the disease [3–8]. Success rates are less than 50% after subchondral collapse has occurred [4,7,8] or in lesions larger than 50% of the femoral head [9,10]. Vascularized fibula grafting has shown superiority over core decompression alone [11] and nonvascularized bone grafting [12]. The procedure; however, is technically difficult and associated with donor site morbidity up to 24% [13,14].

Experience with intertrochanteric or transtrochanteric osteotomies has been variable, with success rates reported from 17% to 91% at short- to mid-term follow-up [15–23]. The clinical success rate of osteotomies decreases when the femoral head lesion combined necrotic angle is greater than 190° [3,16,

24–27]. Conversion to total hip arthroplasty may be difficult after these more conservative procedures.

Therefore, if the osteonecrosis is detected early and the lesion is smaller than 25% to 50% of the femoral head, a bone-preserving operation will have a good chance of achieving long-term success. After subchondral collapse occurs, however, the results of these bone-preserving treatments are less predictable and prosthetic treatments become more appealing. The prosthetic treatment choices include femoral head resurfacing, unipolar or bipolar hemiarthroplasty, and total hip replacement. In young, active patients, the results of any prosthetic treatment are unlikely to last the duration of the patient's lifetime; therefore, the patient is committed to multiple surgical procedures. A conservative prosthetic procedure that preserves bone stock for future surgeries while providing good pain relief and function should be a primary goal of the treating surgeon.

Although unipolar or bipolar hemiarthroplasties initially preserve the acetabular bone stock, the proximal femoral bone is violated for placement of the stem. Results of stemmed hemiarthroplasties are variable, with poor results occurring in over 50% of cases in some series [28–30]. Osteolysis, acetabular protrusio, and stem loosening may add to further bone loss [29,31–33]. If a deep infection occurs, then the resection arthroplasty may be difficult when the stem is still well fixed, leading to additional bone loss.

Total hip arthroplasty usually results in a high rate of initial satisfaction in patients with osteonecrosis; however, long-term results have not been as satisfying compared with the results of other diagnoses. Use of cemented hip replacements for osteonecrosis has resulted in 50% to 92% revision rates at 16 to

E-mail address: mgrecula@utmb.edu

18 years [34,35]. Cementless total hip arthroplasties have yielded lower revision rates of 15% at 11 years [36] but have high rates of osteolysis, stress shielding, and thigh pain [37–39]. Perioperative complications, including dislocation and deep sepsis, have also been shown to be higher in patients with osteonecrosis. When Ortiguera et al [35] compared the results of total hip replacement in osteonecrosis and osteoarthritis, they showed a 7% incidence of dislocation in the osteonecrosis group versus 1% in the osteoarthritis group. Alcohol abuse has also been shown to be associated with a higher dislocation rate [40,41]. Steroid use, systemic lupus erythematosus, sickle cell, and HIV are all associated with higher rates of infection after total hip replacement, with some rates as high as 19% [42–50]. The use of lower-wear bearings or larger heads may hold promise for longer-term durability; however, these results are not yet available.

Experience with resurfacing arthroplasty has been present since the beginning of hip arthroplasty. The evolution in design, materials, and fixation from the original interpositional mold arthroplasty [51] has led to two current resurfacing options for the treatment of osteonecrosis of the femoral head: hemiresurfacing arthroplasty and total resurfacing arthroplasty.

Hemiresurfacing arthroplasty

The hemiresurfacing arthroplasty procedure is the most bone conserving of the arthroplasty options for osteonecrosis. The procedure preserves all of the acetabular bone, the viable portion of the femoral head, and the femoral neck and intramedullary canal. The early series of surface hemiarthroplasties for osteonecrosis included the "adjusted cup" [24], spherocylindric cup [52], or Thomine cup [53]. These were modifications of cup arthroplasties designed to improve fixation to the femoral head without the use of cement. Good and excellent clinical success was seen in 59% to 79% of the cases; however, subluxation, migration, subsidence, and malposition of the cup were commonly seen with these designs.

Townley's [54] description of the total articular replacement arthroplasty (TARA; Depuy, Warsaw, Indiana) procedure recommended removing the proximal third of the femoral head. This bone removal would provide a flat and squared supporting surface of the remaining head, provide maximum mechanical stability and physiologic loading, and remove the bone at risk of vascular compromise. The TARA implant also had a thin, curved stem to aide in precise implant positioning. Scott et al [55]

and Krackow et al [56] reported on the use of the TARA prosthesis for osteonecrosis of the femoral head with good and excellent clinical results in 88% and 84%, respectively. Longer-term follow-up was reported by Hungerford et al [57] who showed 91% survivorship at 5 years and 61% at 10 years. The improved mechanical stability of the implant resulted in a lower complication rate, and only one of the revised implants was noted to be loose.

Amstutz et al [58] performed fixation studies of different femoral component designs and showed that fixation following cylindric reaming was 30% to 50% improved over hemispherical reaming. They believed that the cylindric ream and chamfered contour of the medial femoral head provided a mechanical keying of the component and bone and provided mechanical stability even if a fibrous membrane developed at the bone–cement interface. Using this design with cement fixation, good and excellent results were seen in 83% of the patients at short-term follow-up [59] and a 50% survivorship was reported at 10 years [60]. There were no cases of component loosening or osteolysis, and all of the failures were related to pain.

Several other authors have also reported on their results with hemiresurfacing arthroplasty for osteonecrosis (Table 1). A meta-analysis was performed to further understand the cause of failures for this procedure. Because several of the published results for hemiresurfacing arthroplasty included longer-term follow-up of previously reported cases, only the longer-term follow-up studies of these cases were included for the statistical analysis. Therefore, data were available for 390 patients with 451 surface hemiarthroplasties performed between 1964 and 2000. Of these, 177 were modifications of the cup arthroplasty and placed without cement, whereas 274 of the implants were custom made, the femoral component of a total resurfacing arthroplasty, or designed specifically for hemiresurfacing arthroplasty. The implant material was cobalt-chrome or titanium.

There were 83 complications leading to revision surgery. The most common complication leading to revision surgery was pain related to acetabular cartilage degeneration. This complication accounted for 50 revisions, representing 60% of the revisions and 11% of the series. Subluxation of the cup, absorption of the head under the cup, and migration of the cup were strictly limited to the surface hemiarthroplasties secured without the use of cement. These complications accounted for 17 of the revisions (20%) and 10% of the failures in the cementless hemiarthroplasty group. Nine fractures of the proximal

Table 1
Hemiresurfacing arthroplasty for osteonecrosis

Author, y [Ref.]	No. pts/hips	Age (range)	% Male	Risk factor (%) ST/ETOH/PT/SLE/other	Follow-up (range) (mo)	Good and excellent clinical	No. revisions (%)	Revision reason (no.)
Kerboul et al, 1974 [24]	65/80	—	—	All idiopathic	12–72	66%	13 (16)	3 Neck fracture / 9 Subluxation of cup / 1 Absorption of head
Sedel et al, 1987 [52]	38 hips	40 (17–62)	81	31/31/24/2/12 5% Hemoglobinopathy	83 (12–144)	79%	7 (18)	1 Sepsis / 1 Subluxed cup / 2 Varus cup / 2 Neck resoption and pain / 1 Pain
Tooke et al, 1987 [59] [a]	11/12	31 (20–51)	73	27/46/9/18/0	39 (24–62)	83%	1 (8)	1 Pain
Scott et al, 1987 [55] [a]	20/24	38 (22–55)	90	24/28/16/0/32	37 (25–60)	88%	3 (12.5)	1 Intertrochanteric fracture / 2 Pain
de Meulemeester and Rozing, 1989 [53]	21/27	32 (19–60)	58	57/10/23/0/10	96 (36–144)	—	5 (12.5)	5 Pain
Krackow et al, 1993 [56] [a]	15/19	41 (26–65)	60	60/13/13/0/13	36 (24–72)	84%	3 (16)	—
Amstutz et al, 1994 [60] [a]	9/10	32 (20–51)	78	30/30/10/30/0	114 (40–146)	50%	5 (50)	5 Pain
Nelson et al, 1997 [61]	14/21	33 (18–43)	57	43/19/0/38 19% Sickle cell	74	67%	7 (33)	1 Neck fracture / 6 Pain
Hungerford et al, 1998 [57]	25/33	—	—	26/20/8/26/20	126 (48–168)	61% 82% Excluding SS	13 (39)	1 Femoral loosening / 12 Pain
Beaulé et al, 2001 [65]	33/37	34 (18–51)	81	27/19/35/14/5	75 (22–216)	70%	11 (30)	1 Femoral loosening / 10 Pain
Mont et al, 2001 [66]	30/30	34 (18–57)	60	—	84 (48–101)	—	3 (10)	1 Stem fracture / 1 Dislocation followed by pain
Adili and Trousdale, 2003 [62]	28/29	32 (12–48)	64	43/7/0/14/36	34 (24–63)	62%	8 (28)	6 Pain
Grecula et al, 2004 [64]	67/84	40 (19–66)	47	42/19/5/7/27 2% Hemoglobinopathy 7% HIV	33	60% Pain 80% Walk 77% Function	8 (10)	2 Neck fracture / 6 Pain
Cuckler et al, 2004 [63]	59 pts	38 (19–56)	—	66/17/0/0/17 7% Hemoglobinopathy 2% HIV	53	— / — / —	6 (10)	2 Neck fracture / 4 Pain

Abbreviations: —, data not available; ETOH, alcohol; PT, post-traumatic; pts, patients; SLE, systemic lupus erythematosus; SS, sickle cell; ST, steroid use.
[a] Excluded from analysis.

femur occurred, accounting for 11% of the total failures and a total incidence of 2% in the series. Four of these fractures occurred in the cementless hemiarthroplasty group, one of which occurred in the intertrochanteric region of a patient who underwent radiation therapy for treatment of heterotopic ossification. The other three fractures occurred in the medial portion of the head and were thought to be related to the extension of the necrosis into the inferior part of the head. Five fractures occurred in the cemented hemiarthroplasty group, and all fractures occurred in the subcapital region. Three of these fractures occurred under stemless implants and two occurred with a stemmed implant. One of these fractures occurred in a patient with sickle cell anemia and the other four fractures occurred in femoral heads with lesions greater than 50% of the femoral head. The complications of loosening, migration, subsidence, absorption of the head under the cup, or subluxation of the cup on the head were grouped together because they all represent instability of the cup on the head. These complications were reported in 21 cases, representing 25% of the complications and an incidence of 4.7%. Most cases (19) occurred in the cementless hemiarthroplasties. Loosening was uncommon in the cemented surface hemiarthroplasties (0.7%). There was a low incidence of perioperative complications including dislocation (0.2%), subluxation (0.2%), and sepsis (0.2%) despite a high proportion of patients at risk for perioperative complications after joint arthroplasty because of steroid use, alcohol abuse, systemic lupus erythematosus, or HIV infection.

When failure occurred, the investigators reported that conversion to a total hip arthroplasty was technically as easy as performing a primary total hip arthroplasty and the clinical results of the conversion surgery were equal to the results of primary surgery [57,61–63]. Only four cases of protrusio acetabuli were reported in the series of Thomine cup uncemented hemiarthroplasties [53]. In all the other series, there were no cases of protrusio acetabuli, osteolysis, or significant loss of acetabular or proximal femoral bone stock that complicated the conversion surgery. Narrowing of the articular cartilage space was commonly seen on longer-term follow-up [52,57,61]. During the revision surgery, the acetabulum was characterized by areas of erosion or complete loss of the articular cartilage, and often, the acetabular fossa was filled with bone.

The main disadvantage of hemiresurfacing arthroplasty is the less predictable and sometimes incomplete pain relief. Imperfect sizing was believed to be responsible for an imperfect result in some of the series [24,57]; however, other investigators have not been able to relate sizing of the implant to the clinical outcome [63,64]. Beaulé et al [65] showed an association between the duration of symptoms and acetabular cartilage changes, with a trend to earlier conversion in the hips with longer duration of symptoms; however, this was not statistically significant. Other investigators have also failed to show a predictive relationship of the Ficat stage, preoperative hip score, and duration of symptoms to the clinical outcome [62,63]. In a matched-pair analysis comparing hemiresurfacing arthroplasty to total hip replacement for osteonecrosis, Mont et al [66] showed a higher functional status in patients treated with a hemiresurfacing arthroplasty (60% versus 27%) even though they had a higher incidence of groin pain (20% versus 6%) compared with the total hip replacement group. The ability to predict who will achieve good pain relief after this procedure is difficult and most likely multifactorial. The normal hip joint has been shown to be more of a conchoid shape [67], and the ability to match the normal loading of the articular cartilage may be difficult using a spherical metal head. Other factors affecting pain relief may include the presence of articular cartilage damage, the underlying etiology of the necrosis, and the patients' expectations and response to painful stimuli.

Total resurfacing arthroplasty

Total resurfacing arthroplasty evolved from the double cup arthroplasty and resurfaces both the femoral head and acetabulum. Many authors have reported on their results of total resurfacing arthroplasty, but few have specifically described the results with osteonecrosis. A review of several reported series of total resurfacing arthroplasty shows that the number of procedures performed for osteonecrosis varies from 1% to 36% of the total series [68–73]. The investigators reported a higher loosening rate compared with other diagnoses; however, the number of patients with osteonecrosis in each series was small.

Dutton et al [74] reported on the results of 42 hips in 33 patients who had total hip articular replacement using internal eccentric shells (THARIES; Zimmer, Warsaw, Indiana) cemented surface replacements for osteonecrosis. The patients were followed for an average of 37 months (range, 24–63 months). They reported eight revisions: one for femoral neck fracture, one for sepsis, three for femoral loosening, and three for femoral and acetabular loosening. Radiographic review showed a high percentage of

Table 2
Total resurfacing arthroplasty for osteonecrosis

Author, Y [ref] (Type)	No. pts/hips	No. hips with ON	Age (range)	% Male	Risk factor (%) ST&SLE/ETOH/PT/Other	Average follow-up (mo)	No. revisions (%)	Revision reason
Dutton et al, 1982 [74] (Cemented)	33/42	42	49 (17–64)	64	34/24/24/18	37	8 (19)	1 Neck fracture; 1 Sepsis; 3 Fem loosening; 3 Fem & Acet loosening
de Meulemeester and Rozing, 1989 [53] (Cementless)	11/13	13	37 (22–59)	45	62/15/23/0	96	3 (23)	1 Restricted movement; 1 Dislocation; 1 Varus/protrusion cup
Grecula et al, 1995 [75] (Cemented)	31/35	35	37 (16–50)	86	29/17/26/28	76	19 (54)	2 Neck fracture; 3 Fem loosening; 13 Acet loosening
Grecula et al, 1995 [75] (Cementless)	19/19	19	38 (17–50)	74	11/32/52/5	61	10 (52)	2 Neck fracture; 1 Sepsis; 4 Fem loosening; 1 Fracture acet component; 2 Osteolysis
Beaulé et al, 2004 [76] (Metal/metal hybrid)	56 hips	56	41 (16–56)	82	39/5/25/31	59	3 (5)	2 Fem loosening; 1 Acet loosening
Head, 1981 [70] (Cemented)	40/41	5	—	—	—	29	3 (60)	1 Neck fracture; 1 ON; 1 Fem & acet loosening
Mallory and Danyi, 1982 [73] (Cemented)	44 pts	16	—	—	—	12–31	2 (12.5)	2 Fem loosening
Mallory and Danyi, 1982 [73] (Reverse hybrid)	51 pts	14	—	—	—	12–36	0	—
Jolley et al, 1982 [72] (Cemented)	50/55	10	—	—	—	36	1 (10)	1 Neck fracture
Capello et al, 1984 [68] (Cemented)	96/116	15	—	—	—	24–84	4 (27)	1 ON with fracture; 3 Loosening
Head, 1984 [71] (Reverse hybrid)	63/67	16	—	—	—	40	2 (12.5)	2 Acet loosening

Abbreviations: Acet, acetabular; ETOH, alcohol; Fem, femoral; ON, osteonecrosis; PT, post-traumatic; Pts, patients; ST & SLE, steroid use and systemic lupus erythematosus.

complete acetabular radiolucencies (62%), and the lucencies were greater than 2 mm in 14% of the hips. All of the failures occurred in the 34 hips with nontraumatic osteonecrosis, and the loosening rate, particularly on the femoral side (6 hips), was disappointing. None of the 8 hips with traumatic osteonecrosis experienced failure, and the investigators believed that this may have been related to superior bone quality and less extensive necrosis.

Grecula et al [75] compared the results of cemented total hip replacement, cemented total surface replacement, porous surface replacement, and cemented hemiresurfacing arthroplasty. At 5 years, there was no statistical difference in the survivorship analysis; however, at 8 years, the survivorship of the total surface arthroplasties dropped significantly to 53% for the cemented surface replacement and to 15% for the porous surface replacement, whereas the survivorship of the total hip replacement and hemiresurfacing arthroplasty groups remained satisfactory at 80% and 70%, respectively. Most of the revisions in the total resurfacing groups were related to component loosening or osteolysis, whereas all five of the revisions in the hemiresurfacing group were related to pain without evidence of loosening or osteolysis.

A more recent comparative study between a hybrid metal-on-metal surface arthroplasty versus a cemented hemiresurfacing arthroplasty showed a significant difference between the Harris Hip Scores (92.3 versus 84.1), the physical component scores of the SF-12, and UCLA function and activity scores in favor of the total surface replacement at average of 4.9 years [76]. There was 5% failure of the total surface replacements and 14% failure of the hemiresurfacing arthroplasties; however, the underlying reason for failure was different. In all of the total surface replacements, failure was related to aseptic loosening (two femoral and one acetabular). Three of the four hemiresurfacing arthroplasty failures were related to persistent groin pain, and one was secondary to hematogenous deep sepsis in a patient with Gaucher's disease. The radiographic analysis was also strikingly different, with six of the total surface replacement hips (11%) showing radiographic changes (three femoral lucencies and three neck narrowing), whereas none of the hemiresurfacing arthroplasty hips showed concerning radiographic findings.

A meta-analysis of the available studies on total resurfacing arthroplasty for osteonecrosis was performed to further understand the cause of failures for this procedure (Table 2). To be included in the analysis, the published study needed to include the number of hips with osteonecrosis and provide specific information as to the cause of failure in the

patients with osteonecrosis. If the same author published on the same series, the duplicate series was not included in the analysis. Data were available for 241 hips with osteonecrosis that were treated with total resurfacing arthroplasty performed between 1975 and 2002. One hundred twenty-three procedures used cemented implants, 32 used cementless implants, 56 used hybrid implants (cementless acetabulum and cemented femoral component), and 30 used reverse hybrid implants (cemented acetabulum and cementless femoral component with a stem). The implant material was cobalt-chrome articulating with cobalt-chrome, cobalt-chrome articulating with polyethylene, or titanium articulating with polyethylene. There were 55 (23%) complications leading to revision surgery. The most common complication leading to revision surgery was loosening of one or both of the implants (67% of the revisions, 15% of the series). Acetabular loosening was the most common reason for revision (29%), followed by femoral loosening (27%) and loosening of both implants (11%). Eight femoral neck fractures accounted for 15% of the total failures and a total incidence of 3.3% in the series. Six of these fractures occurred in the cemented group, two in the cementless group, and none in the reverse hybrid group that had a femoral component with a long, curved stem. The femoral neck fracture was believed to originate in an area of osteonecrotic bone in three of the fractures. There was a low incidence of perioperative complications, including dislocation (0.4%) and sepsis (0.8%).

Discussion

The concept of resurfacing the hip joint is appealing because of its bone-conserving nature. On the femoral side, this is true for the hemiresurfacing arthroplasty and total resurfacing arthroplasty procedures. In both procedures, there is minimal resection of the femoral head. During a hemiresurfacing arthroplasty, however, the femoral head does not need to be downsized to allow placement of an acetabular component; therefore, the component size is typically larger and less bone resection is required.

On the acetabular side, the hemiresurfacing arthroplasty is more bone conserving than the total resurfacing procedure in which acetabular bone stock is sacrificed to provide room for an articulating surface. With the older cemented acetabular designs, enough bone had to be removed to accommodate a 4- to 7-mm acetabular component and a cement mantle [77–80]. Less acetabular bone can be removed by downsizing the femoral head to the dimensions of the femoral neck. More recent 3.5-mm cementless acetabular shells with a metal-on-metal bearing reduce the amount of acetabular bone resection to that typically used for a total hip replacement.

In addition to the initial bone preservation related to the conservative femoral cuts, femoral resurfacing has also been shown to preserve the stress distribution to the proximal femur after surgery. Using strain gauge measurements and finite element analysis, Shybut et al [81] showed that the stresses in the distal half of the femoral neck and the remainder of the femoral shaft are unaltered by the presence of the implanted surface replacement hip arthroplasty (THARIES). This study and other studies [82,83]; however, also showed a 50% to 300% increase in the stress concentrations in the lateral/superior and medial/inferior cup-rim region after implantation of a femoral resurfacing implant, which could increase to 500% in osteopenic bone. Recently, a patient-matched study of metal-on-metal surface total hip arthroplasty (Birmingham Hip Resurfacing, Smith and Nephew, Memphis, Tennessee) and total hip replacement with an asymmetric curved titanium alloy (Ti5Al4V) stem (Axcel, Cremascoli, Milan, Italy) showed a significant difference in the bone mineral density of the proximal femoral zones (Gruen zones 1 and 7) [84] at 24 months [85]. The surface replacement femur showed little change in zone 1 and increased density in zone 7 (ratios of 100% and 111%, respectively), whereas the total hip replacement group ratio showed a decrease in density (89% in zone 1 and 83% in zone 7).

Further bone preservation is seen with the hemiresurfacing arthroplasty and is related to the low incidence of acetabular protrusio and periprosthetic osteolysis. Gerard [86] believed that sparing the femoral neck had two advantages over stemmed hemiarthroplasties: (1) the neck length is conserved; therefore, the lever arm through which the gluteus medius acts is preserved; and (2) the forces acting on the hip are transmitted by the bony neck, which retains its normal elasticity. The adverse effect of increased neck length on the articular cartilage has also been demonstrated in a sheep model [87] and may explain the difference in incidence of acetabular protrusio in hemiresurfacing arthroplasty and stemmed hemiarthroplasty. The ability to preserve the femoral head relationships to the femoral shaft, and therefore preserve normal joint relationships and joint mechanics, has also been demonstrated by other investigators [88,89].

The fixation area of the femoral resurfacing component is estimated to be four to five times less than the area available for fixation with an intramedullary stem. The presence of osteonecrotic bone further reduces the available bone surface for fixation. The fixation area can be increased by increasing the size of the component. Mai et al [90] demonstrated a 49% increase in fixation area and a lower incidence of femoral loosening when the larger femoral sizes of the THARIES surface replacement were used. The hemiresurfacing size is limited by the native acetabular size; however, during total resurfacing arthroplasty, a compromise needs to be made between acetabular bone preservation and increasing the femoral fixation area.

Component loosening has been related to inflammatory bone resorption in response to particulate wear debris [91–95]. The absence of an artificial counterbearing in the hemiresurfacing arthroplasty procedure reduces the generation of particulate debris, and there is a lack of osteolysis and neck narrowing noted in retrieval studies [60,61,75]. Therefore, the combined effects of larger fixation area and lack of particulate debris generation may explain the lower incidence of femoral loosening in the hemiresurfacing arthroplasty procedure compared with the total resurfacing arthroplasty results.

The hemiresurfacing arthroplasty and total resurfacing arthroplasty procedures have been successful in reducing the perioperative complications of infection and dislocation to less than 1% despite their use in high-risk patients. The larger femoral head and overall smaller amount of prosthetic material used for surface replacements may account for this difference.

The ability to place a larger femoral component during the hemiresurfacing arthroplasty procedure makes notching the femoral neck less likely and may potentially reduce the risk of femoral neck fracture. The incidence of femoral neck fractures, however, is not significantly different between the hemiresurfacing arthroplasty and total resurfacing arthroplasty groups (2.0% and 3.3%, respectively), which may indicate that the cause of femoral neck fractures is related more to the extent of the necrosis or the stress concentration at the rim of the implant than to the procedure itself. Most investigators do not recommend the procedure when the necrotic area involves more than 30% to 50% of the femoral head [63,68, 74,96].

Further evolution of the necrosis and collapse of the head was believed to be the main cause of failure in one of the cementless hemiresurfacing arthroplasty series [24]; however, progression of the osteonecrosis was not routinely seen in the cemented femoral resurfacing series. Evidence of viable bone has been demonstrated in the femoral head after resurfacing procedures performed for osteonecrosis [60,61,75].

Nelson et al [61] noted peripheral remnants of necrotic bone at the bone cement interface, but the
remainder of the head remained viable. Several other
retrieval studies of femoral heads from failed surface
replacements not specifically performed for osteonecrosis have demonstrated osteonecrosis of the
femoral head associated with femoral neck fractures
in 0.4% to 3.6% of the series [68,72,97–99]. It is not
known whether the necrosis occurred before or after
the femoral neck fracture. Campbell et al [100] noted
necrotic areas in 12% of 25 retrieved femoral heads,
but believed that there was no relation to the cause of
failure. Head [70] reviewed 14 cases of failed Wagner
surface replacements and believed that perioperative
or postoperative necrosis was associated with 7 of the
failures. Therefore, this conflicting information pre-
cludes definite conclusions about the contribution
of perioperative necrosis to the failure of surface
replacements. It is recommended that care be taken

during the procedure to avoid excessive stripping of
the retinacular vessels, to closely observe the vascularity of the femoral head remnant, and to remove
any questionable bone. Preservation of the extramed-
ullary blood supply may not be as critical during
surface replacement for osteoarthritis because the
vascular anastomosis between the metaphysis and
epiphysis may be more developed [101,102].

The approach to the patient with osteonecrosis
needs to be individualized. Multiple factors need to
be considered, including the patient's age and weight,
associated diagnoses and risk factors, comorbidities,
expected activity level, overall expectations of the
procedure, and the size, location, and stage of the
necrotic segment. If the lesion is predicted to have a
low success rate with a head-preserving procedure,
such as core decompression, bone grafting, or osteotomy (large lesions or those that have already
collapsed; Fig. 1A and B), then an arthroplasty

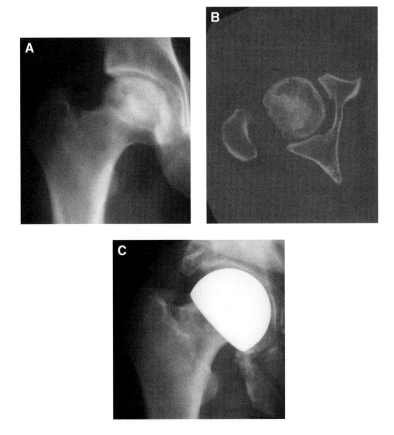

Fig. 1. Thirty-four-year-old white man with bilateral osteonecrosis and history of alcohol use. (*A*) Preoperative radiograph shows
a large necrotic segment with flattening of the femoral head but preserved joint space. (*B*) CT scan shows that the large necrotic
segment extends into the posterior head. The joint space in preserved. (*C*) Radiograph at 9 years postoperatively. The joint space
is still preserved, and the component is stable. The patient is asymptomatic.

solution should be considered. The hemiresurfacing arthroplasty is preferred in young patients or patients with significant comorbidities that would predispose them to a high risk of perioperative complications or loosening with a total hip arthroplasty. The articular cartilage space should be preserved on the radiograph, and there should be minimal changes to the articular cartilage on intraoperative inspection. No exposed subchondral bone and mild fibrillation in only one quadrant should be accepted, although the degree of acetabular cartilage damage is not always predictive of the amount of postoperative pain. The authors also recommend assessing the concentricity of the acetabular fit with trials because often the femoral head is collapsed or deformed, making it difficult to accurately size. The femoral head should have a column of bone that will support a trial implant without a stem, which usually requires at least 50% of the head. The patient should be thoroughly educated on the expectations and limitations of the procedure, mainly the possibility of continued pain and need for another procedure. When successful, enduring results can be obtained with the hemiresurfacing arthroplasty (see Fig. 1C). Total resurfacing has been shown to provide better initial pain relief [76], with the tradeoff of a higher incidence of component loosening, even with the current metal-on-metal bearings designed to produce less particulate debris. Because of the higher incidence of femoral loosening with total resurfacing, more structural femoral head support should be present. When there is more than one-third loss of the femoral head related to the necrosis, the procedure is converted to a total hip arthroplasty using a lower-wear bearing.

References

[1] Mont MA, Carbone JJ, Fairbank AC. Core decompression versus nonoperative management for osteonecrosis of the hip. Clin Orthop 1996;324:169–78.

[2] Etienne G, Mont MA, Ragland PS. The diagnosis and treatment of nontraumatic osteonecrosis of the femoral head. Inst Course Lect 2004;53:67–85.

[3] Ficat RP. Idiopathic bone necrosis of the femoral head: early diagnosis and treatment. J Bone Joint Surg Br 1985;67(1):3–9.

[4] Fairbank AC, Bhatia D, Jinnah RH, et al. Long-term results of core decompression for ischaemic necrosis of the femoral head. J Bone Joint Surg Br 1995; 77(1):42–9.

[5] Koo KH, Kim R, Ko GH, et al. Preventing collapse in early osteonecrosis of the femoral head. A ran-

domised clinical trial of core decompression. J Bone Joint Surg Br 1995;77(6):870–4.

[6] Learmonth ID, Maloon S, Dall G. Core decompression for early atraumatic osteonecrosis of the femoral head. J Bone Joint Surg Br 1990;72(3):387–90.

[7] Lausten GS, Mathiesen B. Core decompression for femoral head necrosis. Prospective study of 28 patients. Acta Orthop Scand 1990;61(6):507–11.

[8] Smith SW, Fehring TK, Griffin WL, et al. Core decompression of the osteonecrotic femoral head. J Bone Joint Surg Am 1995;77(5):674–80.

[9] Beltran J, Knight CT, Zuelzer WA, et al. Core decompression for avascular necrosis of the femoral head: correlation between long-term results and preoperative MR staging. Radiology 1990;175(2): 533–6.

[10] Holman AJ, Gardner GC, Richardson ML, et al. Quantitative magnetic resonance imaging predicts clinical outcome of core decompression for osteonecrosis of the femoral head. J Rheumatol 1995;22(10): 1929–33.

[11] Kane SM, Ward WA, Jordan LC, et al. Vascularized fibular grafting compared with core decompression in the treatment of femoral head osteonecrosis. Orthopedics 1996;19(10):869–72.

[12] Plakseychuk AY, Kim SY, Park BC, et al. Vascularized compared with nonvascularized fibular grafting for the treatment of osteonecrosis of the femoral head. J Bone Joint Surg Am 2003;85(4):589–96.

[13] Vail TP, Urbaniak JR. Donor-site morbidity with use of vascularized autogenous fibular grafts. J Bone Joint Surg Am 1996;78(2):204–11.

[14] Urbaniak JR, Harvey EJ. Revascularization of the femoral head in osteonecrosis. J Am Acad Orthop Surg 1998;6(1):44–54.

[15] Ganz R, Buchler U. Overview of attempts to revitalize the dead head in aseptic necrosis of the femoral head: osteotomy and revascularization. In: Hungerford DS, editor. The hip: proceedings of the 11th Open Scientific Meeting of the Hip Society. St. Louis (MO): Mosby; 1983. p. 296–305.

[16] Mont MA, Fairbank AC, Krackow KA, et al. Corrective osteotomy for osteonecrosis of the femoral head. J Bone Joint Surg Am 1996;78(7):1032–8.

[17] Ito H, Kaneda K, Matsuno T. Osteonecrosis of the femoral head. Simple varus intertrochanteric osteotomy. J Bone Joint Surg Br 1999;81(6):969–74.

[18] Pavlovcic V, Dolinar D. Intertrochanteric osteotomy for osteonecrosis of the femoral head. Int Orthop 2002;26(4):238–42.

[19] Sugioka Y, Hotokebuchi T, Tsutsui H. Transtrochanteric anterior rotational osteotomy for idiopathic and steroid-induced necrosis of the femoral head. Indications and long-term results. Clin Orthop 1992; 277:111–20.

[20] Sugano N, Takaoka K, Ohzono K, et al. Rotational osteotomy for non-traumatic avascular necrosis of the femoral head. J Bone Joint Surg Br 1992;74(5): 734–9.

[21] Inao S, Ando M, Gotoh E, et al. Minimum 10-year results of Sugioka's osteotomy for femoral head osteonecrosis. Clin Orthop 1999;368:141–8.

[22] Grigoris P, Safran M, Brown I, et al. Long-term results of transtrochanteric rotational osteotomy for femoral head osteonecrosis. Arch Orthop Trauma Surg 1996;115(3–4):127–30.

[23] Dean MT, Cabanela ME. Transtrochanteric anterior rotational osteotomy for avascular necrosis of the femoral head. Long-term results. J Bone Joint Surg Br 1993;75(4):597–601.

[24] Kerboul M, Thomine J, Postel M, et al. The conservative surgical treatment of idiopathic aseptic necrosis of the femoral head. J Bone Joint Surg Br 1974;56(2):291–6.

[25] Jacobs MA, Hungerford DS, Krackow KA. Intertrochanteric osteotomy for avascular necrosis of the femoral head. J Bone Joint Surg Br 1989;71(2):200–4.

[26] Santore RF. Intertrochanteric osteotomy for osteonecrosis. Semin Arthroplasty 1991;2(3):208–13.

[27] Dinulescu I, Stanculescu D, Nicolescu M, et al. Long-term follow-up after intertrochanteric osteotomies for avascular necrosis of the femoral head. Bull Hosp Joint Dis 1998;57(2):84–7.

[28] Beckenbaugh RD, Tressler HA, Johnson Jr EW. Results after hemiarthroplasty of the hip using a cemented femoral prosthesis. A review of 109 cases with an average follow-up of 36 months. Mayo Clin Proc 1977;52(6):349–53.

[29] Lachiewicz PF, Desman SM. The bipolar endoprosthesis in avascular necrosis of the femoral head. J Arthroplasty 1988;3(2):131–8.

[30] Ito H, Matsuno T, Kaneda K. Bipolar hemiarthroplasty for osteonecrosis of the femoral head. A 7- to 18-year follow up. Clin Orthop 2000;374:201–11.

[31] Takaoka K, Nishina T, Ohzono K, et al. Bipolar prosthetic replacement for the treatment of avascular necrosis of the femoral head. Clin Orthop 1992;277:121–7.

[32] Kim KJ, Rubash HE. Large amounts of polyethylene debris in the interface tissue surrounding bipolar endoprostheses. Comparison to total hip prostheses. J Arthroplasty 1997;12(1):32–9.

[33] Cabanela ME. The bipolar prosthesis in avascular necrosis of the femoral head. Semin Arthroplasty 1991;2(3):228–33.

[34] Dorr LD, Kane III TJ, Conaty JP. Long-term results of cemented total hip arthroplasty in patients 45 years old or younger: a 16-year follow-up study. J Arthroplasty 1994;9(5):453–6.

[35] Ortiguera CJ, Pulliam IT, Cabanela ME. Total hip arthroplasty for osteonecrosis: matched-pair analysis of 188 hips with long-term follow-up. J Arthroplasty 1999;14(1):21–8.

[36] Kim YH, Kim JS, Cho SH. Primary total hip arthroplasty with the AML total hip prosthesis. Clin Orthop 1999;360:147–58.

[37] Kim YH, Oh JH, Oh SH. Cementless total hip arthroplasty in patients with osteonecrosis of the femoral head. Clin Orthop 1995;320:73–84.

[38] Piston RW, Engh CA, De Carvalho PI, et al. Osteonecrosis of the femoral head treated with total hip arthroplasty without cement. J Bone Joint Surg Am 1994;76(2):202–14.

[39] Kim YH, Oh SH, Kim JS, et al. Contemporary total hip arthroplasty with and without cement in patients with osteonecrosis of the femoral head. J Bone Joint Surg Am 2003;85(4):675–81.

[40] Paterno SA, Lachiewicz PF, Kelley SS. The influence of patient-related factors and the position of the acetabular component on the rate of dislocation after total hip replacement. J Bone Joint Surg Am 1997;79(8):1202–10.

[41] Espehaug B, Havelin LI, Engesaeter LB, et al. Patient-related risk factors for early revision of total hip replacements. A population register-based case-control study of 674 revised hips. Acta Orthop Scand 1997;68(3):207–15.

[42] Phillips FM, Pottenger LA, Finn HA, et al. Cementless total hip arthroplasty in patients with steroid-induced avascular necrosis of the hip. A 62-month follow-up study. Clin Orthop 1994;303:147–54.

[43] Zangger P, Gladman DD, Urowitz MB, et al. Outcome of total hip replacement for avascular necrosis in systemic lupus erythematosus. J Rheumatol 2000;27(4):919–23.

[44] Hanssen AD, Cabanela ME, Michet CJ. Hip arthroplasty in patients with systemic lupus erythematosus. J Bone Joint Surg Am 1987;69(6):807–14.

[45] Al Mousawi F, Malki A, Al Aradi A, et al. Total hip replacement in sickle cell disease. Int Orthop 2002;26(3):157–61.

[46] Ilyas I, Moreau P. Simultaneous bilateral total hip arthroplasty in sickle cell disease. J Arthroplasty 2002;17(4):441–5.

[47] Parvizi J, Sullivan TA, Pagnano MW, et al. Total joint arthroplasty in human immunodeficiency virus-positive patients: an alarming rate of early failure. J Arthroplasty 2003;18(3):259–64.

[48] Kelley SS, Lachiewicz PF, Gilbert MS, et al. Hip arthroplasty in hemophilic arthropathy. J Bone Joint Surg Am 1995;77(6):828–34.

[49] Hicks JL, Ribbans WJ, Buzzard B, et al. Infected joint replacements in HIV-positive patients with haemophilia. J Bone Joint Surg Br 2001;83(7):1050–4.

[50] Lehman CR, Ries MD, Paiement GD, et al. Infection after total joint arthroplasty in patients with human immunodeficiency virus or intravenous drug use. J Arthroplasty 2001;16(3):330–5.

[51] Smith-Petersen MN. Evolution of mould arthroplasty of the hip joint. J Bone Joint Surg Br 1948;30(1):59–75.

[52] Sedel L, Travers V, Witvoet J. Spherocylindric (Luck) cup arthroplasty for osteonecrosis of the hip. Clin Orthop 1987;219:127–35.

[53] de Meulemeester FR, Rozing PM. Uncemented sur-

face replacement for osteonecrosis of the femoral head. Acta Orthop Scand 1989;60(4):425–9.

[54] Townley CO. Hemi and total articular replacement arthroplasty of the hip with the fixed femoral cup. Orthop Clin N Am 1982;13(4):869–94.

[55] Scott RD, Urse JS, Schmidt R, et al. Use of TARA hemiarthroplasty in advanced osteonecrosis. J Arthroplasty 1987;2(3):225–32.

[56] Krackow KA, Mont MA, Maar DC. Limited femoral endoprosthesis for avascular necrosis of the femoral head. Orthop Rev 1993;22(4):457–63.

[57] Hungerford MW, Mont MA, Scott R, et al. Surface replacement hemiarthroplasty for the treatment of osteonecrosis of the femoral head. J Bone Joint Surg Am 1998;80(11):1656–64.

[58] Amstutz HC, Clarke IC, Christie J, et al. Total hip articular replacement by internal eccentric shells: the "tharies" approach to total surface replacement arthroplasty. Clin Orthop 1977;128:261–84.

[59] Tooke SM, Amstutz HC, Delaunay C. Hemiresurfacing for femoral head osteonecrosis. J Arthroplasty 1987;2(2):125–33.

[60] Amstutz HC, Grigoris P, Safran MR, et al. Precision-fit surface hemiarthroplasty for femoral head osteonecrosis: long-term results. J Bone Joint Surg Br 1994;76(3):423–7.

[61] Nelson CL, Walz BH, Gruenwald JM. Resurfacing of only the femoral head for osteonecrosis: Long-term follow-up study. J Arthroplasty 1997;12(7):736–40.

[62] Adili A, Trousdale RT. Femoral head resurfacing for the treatment of osteonecrosis in the young patient. Clin Orthop 2003;417:93–101.

[63] Cuckler JM, Moore DK, Estrada L. Outcome of hemiresurfacing in osteonecrosis of the femoral head. Clin Orthop 2004;429(429):146–50.

[64] Grecula MJ, Thomas JA, Kreuzer SW. Impact of implant design on femoral head hemiresurfacing arthroplasty. Clin Orthop 2004;418:41–7.

[65] Beaulé PE, Schmalzried TP, Campbell P, et al. Duration of symptoms and outcome of hemiresurfacing for hip osteonecrosis. Clin Orthop 2001;385:104–17.

[66] Mont MA, Rajadhyaksha AD, Hungerford DS. Outcomes of limited femoral resurfacing arthroplasty compared with total hip arthroplasty for osteonecrosis of the femoral head. J Arthroplasty 2001;16(8 Suppl 1):134–9.

[67] Menschik F. The hip joint as a conchoid shape. J Biomech 1997;30(9):971–3.

[68] Capello WN, Misamore GW, Trancik TM. The Indiana conservative (surface-replacement) hip arthroplasty. J Bone Joint Surg Am 1984;66(4):518–28.

[69] Freeman MA, Bradley GW. ICLH surface replacement of the hip. An analysis of the first 10 years. J Bone Joint Surg Br 1983;65(4):405–11.

[70] Head WC. Wagner surface replacement arthroplasty of the hip. Analysis of fourteen failures in forty-one hips. J Bone Joint Surg Am 1981;63(3):420–7.

[71] Head WC. Total articular resurfacing arthroplasty.

Analysis of component failure in sixty-seven hips. J Bone Joint Surg Am 1984;66(1):28–34.

[72] Jolley MN, Salvati EA, Brown GC. Early results and complications of surface replacement of the hip. J Bone Joint Surg Am 1982;64(3):366–77.

[73] Mallory TH, Danyi J. Conservative total hip replacement. Orthopedics 1982;5(8):1012–5.

[74] Dutton RO, Amstutz HC, Thomas BJ, et al. Tharies surface replacement for osteonecrosis of the femoral head. J Bone Joint Surg Am 1982;64(8):1225–37.

[75] Grecula MJ, Grigoris P, Schmalzried TP, et al. Endoprostheses for osteonecrosis of the femoral head. A comparison of four models in young patients. Int Orthop 1995;19(3):137–43.

[76] Beaulé PE, Amstutz HC, Le Duff M, et al. Surface arthroplasty for osteonecrosis of the hip: hemiresurfacing versus metal-on-metal hybrid resurfacing. J Arthroplasty 2004;19(8 Suppl 3):54–8.

[77] Amstutz HC, Graff-Radford A, Gruen TA, et al. THARIES surface replacements: a review of the first 100 cases. Clin Orthop 1978;134:87–101.

[78] Wagner H. Surface replacement arthroplasty of the hip. Clin Orthop 1978;134:102–30.

[79] Freeman MA, Cameron HU, Brown GC. Cemented double cup arthroplasty of the hip: a 5 year experience with the ICLH prosthesis. Clin Orthop 1978;134:45–52.

[80] Trentani C, Vaccarino F. The Paltrinieri-Trentani hip joint resurface arthroplasty. Clin Orthop 1978;134:36–40.

[81] Shybut GT, Askew MJ, Horii RY, et al. Theoretical and experimental studies of femoral stresses following surface replacement hip arthroplasty. In: Riley Jr LH, editor. The hip: proceedings of the 8th Open Scientific Meeting of the Hip Society. St. Louis (MO): C.V. Mosby; 1980. p. 192–224.

[82] Watanabe Y, Shiba N, Matsuo S, et al. Biomechanical study of the resurfacing hip arthroplasty: finite element analysis of the femoral component. J Arthroplasty 2000;15(4):505–11.

[83] Huiskes R, Strens PH, van Heck J, et al. Interface stresses in the resurfaced hip. Finite element analysis of load transmission in the femoral head. Acta Orthop Scand 1985;56(6):474–8.

[84] Gruen TA, McNeice GM, Amstutz HC. "Modes of failure" of cemented stem-type femoral components: a radiographic analysis of loosening. Clin Orthop 1979;141:17–27.

[85] Kishida Y, Sugano N, Nishii T, et al. Preservation of the bone mineral density of the femur after surface replacement of the hip. J Bone Joint Surg Br 2004;86(2):185–9.

[86] Gerard Y. Hip arthroplasty by matching cups. Clin Orthop 1978;134:25–35.

[87] van der Meulen MC, Beaupre GS, Smith RL, et al. Factors influencing changes in articular cartilage following hemiarthroplasty in sheep. J Orthop Res 2002;20(4):669–75.

[88] Amstutz HC, Beaulé PE, Dorey FJ, et al. Metal-

on-metal hybrid surface arthroplasty: two to six-year follow-up study. J Bone Joint Surg Am 2004;86(1): 28–39.

[89] Silva M, Lee KH, Heisel C, et al. The biomechanical results of total hip resurfacing arthroplasty. J Bone Joint Surg Am 2004;86(1):40–6.

[90] Mai MT, Schmalzried TP, Dorey FJ, et al. The contribution of frictional torque to loosening at the cement-bone interface in Tharies hip replacements. J Bone Joint Surg Am 1996;78(4):505–11.

[91] Amstutz HC, Campbell P, Kossovsky N, et al. Mechanism and clinical significance of wear debris-induced osteolysis. Clin Orthop 1992;276:7–18.

[92] Howie DW, Cornish BL, Vernon-Roberts B. Resurfacing hip arthroplasty. Classification of loosening and the role of prosthesis wear particles. Clin Orthop 1990;255:144–59.

[93] Nasser S, Campbell PA, Kilgus D, et al. Cementless total joint arthroplasty prostheses with titanium-alloy articular surfaces. A human retrieval analysis. Clin Orthop 1990;261:171–85.

[94] Santavirta S, Hoikka V, Eskola A, et al. Aggressive granulomatous lesions in cementless total hip arthroplasty. J Bone Joint Surg Br 1990;72(6): 980–4.

[95] Schmalzried TP, Jasty M, Harris WH. Peripros-thetic bone loss in total hip arthroplasty. Polyethylene wear debris and the concept of the effective joint space. J Bone Joint Surg Am 1992;74(6): 849–63.

[96] Shea WD. Indications and contraindications in surface replacement arthroplasty of the hip. Orthop Clin N Am 1982;13(4):729–37.

[97] Bell RS, Schatzker J, Fornasier VL, et al. A study of implant failure in the Wagner resurfacing arthroplasty. J Bone Joint Surg Am 1985;67(8):1165–75.

[98] Bradley GW, Freeman MA, Revell PA. Resurfacing arthroplasty. Femoral head viability. Clin Orthop 1987;220:137–41.

[99] Bogoch ER, Fornasier VL, Capello WN. The femoral head remnant in resurfacing arthroplasty. Clin Orthop 1982;167:92–105.

[100] Campbell P, Mirra J, Amstutz HC. Viability of femoral heads treated with resurfacing arthroplasty. J Arthroplasty 2000;15(1):120–2.

[101] Freeman MA. Some anatomical and mechanical considerations relevant to the surface replacement of the femoral head. Clin Orthop 1978;134:19–24.

[102] Whiteside LA, Lange DR, Capello WR, et al. The effects of surgical procedures on the blood supply to the femoral head. J Bone Joint Surg Am 1983; 65(8):1127–33.

ELSEVIER
SAUNDERS

Orthop Clin N Am 36 (2005) 243–250

ORTHOPEDIC
CLINICS
OF NORTH AMERICA

Clinical Correlation of Femoral Component Migration in Hip Resurfacing Arthroplasty Analyzed by Einzel-Bild-Röntgen-Analyze–Femoral Component Analysis

Vincent A. Fowble, MD[a], Alexander Schuh, MD[b], Ryan Hoke, BS[a],
Rudi G. Bitsch, MD[a], Paul E. Beaulé, MD, FRCSC[a,c,*]

[a]Joint Replacement Institute at Orthopaedic Hospital, 2400 S. Flower Street, Los Angeles, CA 90007, USA
[b]Orthopedic Clinic Wichernhaus, 90592 Schwarzenbruck, Germany
[c]Department of Orthopaedics, David Geffen School of Medicine at University of California Los Angeles, 1250 16th Street, Suite 745, Los Angeles, CA 90404, USA

Hip resurfacing arthroplasty has gained a renewed interest because of advances in new bearing technology, with metal-on-metal bearing designs being implanted throughout Europe and Australia and current clinical trials underway in the United States. As a beneficial solution for active, young adults with osteoarthritis of the hip, this interest has been pursued due to hip resurfacing's bone-preserving characteristics, anatomic reconstruction with more normal stress transfer to the proximal femur, and ease for conversion to a total hip arthroplasty [1–6].

Metal-on-metal bearings have shown a significant decrease in volumetric wear, with no apparent "wear penalty" with the larger-diameter surface replacements [7]. The wear of a metal-on-metal bearing is imperceptible on plain radiographs; thus, migration analysis studies may represent the opportunity to detect early failures and evaluate long-term prosthetic survival [8]. Several studies have correlated early femoral component migration at 2 years and failure in total hip arthroplasty [9–13]. There are different methods to detect femoral component migration. Roentgen stereophotogrammetric analysis and Einzel-Bild-Röntgen-Analyze (EBRA) have been described [9,14–17]. Roentgen stereophotogrammetric analysis has been the most accurate method; however, it involves the implantation of tantalum markers at the time of surgery, with the associated increased cost and possibility of third-body particles being introduced. Beaulé et al [14] recently tested and validated an EBRA method for evaluating femoral component migration in hip resurfacing arthroplasty. They found that EBRA femoral component analysis (EBRA-FCA) was reliable and demonstrated an accuracy of 1.6 mm in the x-axis and 2.0 mm in the y-axis.

The purpose of the present study was to retrospectively analyze the femoral component migration by means of EBRA-FCA in a consecutive series of metal-on-metal surface arthroplasty of the hip with long-term clinical follow-up.

Materials and methods

Between November 1993 and July 1996, 42 McMinn (Corin Medical, Cirencester, United Kingdom) cemented surface arthroplasties of the hip were performed in 41 patients (1 bilateral). The early (average,

---

* Corresponding author. Joint Replacement Institute at Orthopaedic Hospital, 2400 S. Flower Street, Los Angeles, CA 90007.

E-mail address: pbeaule@laoh.ucla.edu (H.C. Beaulé).

0030-5898/05/$ – see front matter © 2005 Elsevier Inc. All rights reserved.
doi:10.1016/j.ocl.2005.02.008

16 months) and intermediate (average, 8.7 years) clinical results of this series of McMinn surface replacements have been published [4,18]. Currently, at an average of 9 years of follow-up, 16 of the 42 hips have been revised. The primary mode of failure was in the acetabulum, with 11 hips requiring revision due to dissociation of the acetabular cup– cement interface and 1 hip having aseptic loosening of a cementless acetabular component. There were 2 hips with femoral component loosening, 1 with femoral neck fracture, and 1 case of sepsis.

The EBRA-FCA software for hip resurfacing arthroplasty [14] was used to analyze these cases using anteroposterior radiographs that had been obtained in a nonstandardized fashion. Twenty-nine hips (28 patients) with a mean follow-up of 93.8 months (range, 46.8–123.8 months) composed the study group. This group included 12 of the 16 hips requiring a revision procedure. Thirteen hips (13 patients) were excluded from the study. The exclusions included 3 hips in 3 patients lost to follow-up (1 of these hips was revised by an outside surgeon); 2 hips in 2 patients who sustained subtrochanteric femur fractures (not related to the surgery); 1 hip that was revised for femoral neck fracture at 9.7 months, 1 hip lost due to patient death (secondary to unrelated causes) within the first year following the operation, 1 hip that developed a septic joint, and 5 hips in 5 patients who had inadequate or low-quality radiographs rejected by the EBRA analysis. The patient demographics and etiologies for the 29 hips are presented in Table 1.

The accuracy of the EBRA-FCA program is perceived by a comparability strategy of radiographs. Defined reference lines in the x-axis and y-axis of the radiographs within a series of radiographs of the same patient are compared with each other. Migration is measured only between pairs of radiographs with comparable reference lines of the prosthesis, whereas the others are excluded from the measurements. The comparability limit was 2 mm [14,17].

For EBRA analysis, all available radiographs used were scanned into a digital format and analyzed by the EBRA-FCA software program. In the revision cases, the latest radiograph before the revision surgery was scanned and analyzed by EBRA-FCA. On average, there were 10 consecutive radiographs per patient per series available for EBRA-FCA analysis. Due to the comparability algorithm of the software, 47% of radiographs were excluded from calculation of migration (not comparable with the other radiographs of a series). The authors particularly focused on the EBRA findings within the first 2 years following implantation and how they correlated with the known clinical outcomes as reported by Beaulé

Table 1
Demographics and etiologies (N = 29)

	Mean	SD	Range	n
Demographics				
Age at surgery (y)	45.7	12.1	22.5–67.8	
Weight (kg)	76.9	19.8	39.0–118.0	
Height (cm)	166.1	6.7	148–198	
Male/female patients	14/15			
Charnley class A/B/C	10/15/4			
SARI	3	1.8	0–6	
Etiology				
Osteoarthritis				13
Osteonecrosis				6
Developmental dysplasia				3
Arthrokatadysis				2
Legg-Calvé-Perthes				1
Slipped capital femoral epiphysis				2
Rheumatoid arthritis				1
Juvenile rheumatoid arthritis				1

Abbreviation: SARI, surface arthroplasty risk index [20].

et al [14]. All patients were evaluated clinically using the University of California Los Angeles hip score for pain, walking, function, and activity [19] and by radiographic examination with anteroposterior pelvis and Johnson-lateral radiographs. Femoral components with a stem lucency >1 mm were considered loose [20]. Implant retrieval analysis was performed on five available femoral components and evaluated according to the grading system set forth by Howie et al [21] in assessing the degree of loosening. These grades included grade 0: well fixed with intact bone– cement contact; grade 1: fixed with connective tissue–cement contact; grade 2: slightly loose, with possible necrosis or apparent surface abrasion; and grade 3: markedly loose with loss of femoral head shape and significant bone loss. Migration patterns as measured by EBRA-FCA were then correlated with hips with femoral component failure defined as stem lucency >1 mm, component condition at time of revision surgery, and implant retrieval analysis. Attention was directed to the two cases of known femoral loosening (at time of revision) and any cases in which EBRA showed significant migration. Overall migrations of 2 mm were considered detectable migrations within the comparability limits between radiographs. Overall migration was defined as the magnitude (expressed in millimeters) of the migration vector sum along the x-axis and the y-axis for the given points of interest, the head center, and the stem tip.

Table 2
Group I: femoral components with migration at 2 years

Group	Case	Hip no.	Net head migration at 2-y FU	Overall tip migration at 2-y FU	No. of radiographs	Time to last radiography analyzed (mo)	Net head migration at LFU	Overall tip migration at LFU	MFU	Stem lucency size (mm)	Revised	MREV	Femoral component loosening	UCLA score at LFU P	W	F	A
Group I-A[a]																	
	1	7	3.35	0.72	4	82.6	2.60	1.41		2	Yes	88.1	Yes				
	2	31	3.62	1.90	7	67.9	5.60	3.20		9	Yes	81.4	Yes				
	3	16	1.84	2.28	4	84.0	1.84	2.28		8	Yes	93.2	Yes				
	4	18	6.16	5.71	8	95.2	7.96	7.55	106.1	3	No		Probable	10	10	8	6
	5	15	3.05	1.63	10	108.0	3.38	1.36	119.5	0	No		No	9	8	8	7
Average			3.6	2.4	6.6	87.5	4.3	3.2				87.6					
Group I-B[b]																	
	6	21	5.46	4.79	4	67.9	0.81	1.58		0	Yes	71.1	No	9	9	9	6
	7	4	2.89	1.41	3	101.6	1.90	0.50	102.4	0	No		No	10	9	10	6
	8	13	2.62	1.94	5	41.0	1.64	1.17	89.1	0	No		No	10	9	10	9
	9	22	2.64	2.55	8	93.9	1.28	0.94	94.6	0	No		No	8	10	10	7
	10	23	3.54	0.32	8	85.7	1.68	1.02	90.3	1	No		No	10	10	10	7
	11	36	2.58	2.08	7	102.7	1.17	0.64	102.8	0	No		No				
Average			3.29	2.18	6.22	82.13	1.41	0.98	95.84					9.4	9.6	9.8	7
Group I average			3.43	2.30	6.18	84.59	2.71	1.97	100.69			83.45		9.4	9.4	9.3	6.9

Abbreviations: A, activity; F, function; FU, follow-up; LFU, latest follow-up; MFU, months to follow-up; MREV, months to revision; P, pain; W, walking.
[a] Femoral components with migration at LFU.
[b] Femoral components without migration at LFU.

Table 3

Group II: femoral components with no migration at 2 years

Group	Case	Hip no.	Net head migration at 2-y FU	Overall tip migration at 2-y FU	No. of radiographs	Time to last radiograph analyzed (mo)	Net head migration at LFU	Overall tip migration at LFU	MFU	Stem lucency size (mm)	Revised	MREV	Femoral component loosening	UCLA score at LFU P	W	F	A
Group II-A[a]																	
	12	9	0.94	0.63	5	62.3	2.30	1.20	82.0	0			No	10	10	10	4
	13	27	0.45	0.14	7	84.0	4.26	0.58	88.6	0			No	8	10	10	7
	14	32	1.39	0.78	7	86.7	2.18	1.04	110.3	0			No	10	4	4	3
	15	30	0.71	0.63	6	62.0	6.67	5.36	62.1	0			No	10	10	4	4
	16	35	0.00	0.00	3	98.1	5.28	1.94	98.6	2			Probable	8	9	9	6
	17	12	1.90	0.98	9	115.3	1.92	4.93	115.3	3.5			Probable	9	8	6	5
	18	29	1.80	1.25	4	109.4	3.52	4.73		1.5	Yes	113.2	Yes	9	10	10	8
	19	6	0.36	0.32	6	62.4	4.60	4.20		1.5	Yes	123.8	Yes				
Average			0.94	0.59	5.875	85.03	3.84	3.00	92.82					9.14	8.7	7.6	5.3
Group II-B[b]																	
	20	2	0.51	0.54	8	94.7	1.14	1.24		0.5	Yes	95.5	No	10	8	8	5
	21	20	1.98	0.98	7	106.0	0.45	0.30		0	Yes	106.3	No				
	22	25	0.10	0.36	5	35.2	0.10	0.36		0.5	Yes	46.8	No				
	23	3	1.55	0.76	6	106.5	1.55	0.76	106.5	1	Yes	25.1	No-retained	9	10	10	7
	24	8	1.00	1.06	6	96.9	0.85	1.34	96.9	0	Yes	24.9	No-retained	10	10	9	8
	25	10	1.43	1.80	10	84.9	1.61	1.63	85.0	1	Yes	26.5	No-retained	7	9	8	6
Average									96.1								
	26	14	0.91	1.99	6	57.0	0.32	1.12	96.3	0	No		No	10	10	10	9
	27	34	0.00	0.00	3	69.3	1.14	1.10	81.1	0	No		No	10	10	8	5
	28	38	1.90	0.71	5	92.1	1.90	0.86	92.1	0.5	No		No	6	4	4	4
	29	33	1.41	0.85	7	80.5	1.00	0.85	80.5	2	No		Probable	9	10	10	10
Average			1.08	0.91	6.30	82.31	1.03	0.96	90.69			54.2		8.88	8.9	8.4	6.8
Group II average			1.02	0.77	6.11	83.52	2.28	1.86	91.95			70.24		9	8.8	8	6.1

Abbreviations: A, activity; F, function; FU, follow-up; LFU, latest follow-up; MFU, months to follow-up; MREV, months to revision; P, pain; W, walking.

[a] Femoral components with migration at LFU.

[b] Femoral components without migration at LFU.

Table 4
Sensitivity and specificity

Migration at follow-up	FC loose or RL >1 mm (n)	Clinically functional and RL ≤1 mm (n)
Migration at 2 y	4[a]	7[b]
No migration at 2 y	5[a]	13[b]
Migration at LFU	8[c]	5[d]
No migration at LFU	1[c]	15[d]

Abbreviations: FC, femoral component; LFU, latest follow-up; RL, radiolucency.

[a] Sensitivity: 4/9 = 0.444.
[b] Specificity: 13/20 = 0.65.
[c] Sensitivity: 8/9 = 0.888.
[d] Specificity: 15/20 = 0.75.

Analysis of variance was used to compare the difference in magnitude of migration patterns, specifically looking at the maximum absolute value of change in migration at the stem tip or the femoral head. The 95% confidence intervals (CI) were used.

Results

EBRA analysis of the 29 hips revealed femoral component migration greater than 2 mm in 11 hips (group I) at the 2-year analysis (Table 2). The average migration was 3.43 mm for the center of the femoral head and 2.30 mm for the stem tip. Clinically, 4 of 11 hips were revised at an average of 83.5 months (range, 71–93 months). The remaining 7 hips that have not been revised remain clinically functional at an average of 100.7 months (range, 89–119 months) (see Table 2). Of the 4 revised hips, 2 hips (cases 2 and 3) were revised for femoral component loosening at outside facilities. The other 2 hips (cases 1 and 6) were revised for acetabular cup–cement interface dissociation. Implant retrieval analysis for these two femoral components indicated that one femoral component (case 1) was slightly loose (grade 2.3), which corresponded with a 2-mm radiolucency seen on radiograph and a more subtle migration pattern by EBRA-FCA at latest follow-up, and the other femoral component (case 6) was stable and well fixed (grade 0), which corresponded with no radiolucency noted on radiograph and no migration at latest follow-up.

Group I was further divided into two groups based on latest follow-up migration patterns. Group I-A (five hips) demonstrated migration, whereas group I-B (six hips) did not. Two hips within group I-A (cases 4 and 5), which remain clinically functional, continued to show migration at latest follow-up; one of these hips (case 4) demonstrated significant migration of the femoral head and stem tip and was associated with a 3-mm radiolucency. This hip was designated as loose. The other hip (case 5) within group I-A showed femoral head migration but no stem tip migration and no associated radiolucencies. This hip was deemed stable. The remaining three hips in group I-A (cases 1–3) were revised as stated earlier. The other five hips were within group I-B and showed no migration at latest follow-up and no radiolucencies >1 mm. The sixth hip (case 6) was revised as stated earlier.

Eighteen of the 29 hips (group II) showed no migration detected by EBRA-FCA analysis at the 2-year interval (Table 3). Within group II, 8 hips were revised at an average of 70.2 months (range, 24–123 months) and the remaining 10 are clinically functioning well at an average of 90.7 months (range, 62–115 months). Group II was further subdivided into group II-A and group II-B. Group II-A included 8 hips with a detected migration (average, 3.84 mm for the center of the femoral head and 3.00 mm for the stem tip) at latest follow-up and group II-B included 10 hips with no migration detected by EBRA-FCA. Within group II-A, 4 hips (cases 16–19) had stem lucencies >1 mm and were designated as

Table 5
Migration patterns

| Migration patterns | At 2 y | | At LFU | |
	Femoral component loose	Femoral component not loose	Femoral component loose	Femoral component not loose
Femoral head and stem tip <2 mm	5	13	1	15
Femoral head >2 mm, stem tip <2 mm	2	4	2	4
Femoral head <2 mm, stem tip >2 mm	1	0	2	0
Femoral head and stem tip >2 mm	1	3	4	1

Abbreviation: LFU, latest follow-up.

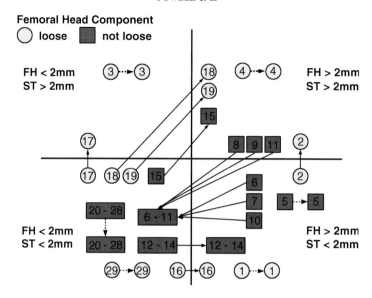

Fig. 1. Schematic representing the four different migration patterns in a quadrant coordinate axis. Each case is represented by a circle (femoral component loose) or a square (femoral component not loose), with a vector arrow indicating the changing migration pattern seen between the 2-year and latest follow-up analysis. FH, femoral head; ST, stem tip.

loose; cases 18 and 19 were revised for acetabular component failure and implant retrieval analysis confirmed femoral loosening. Within group II-B, 6 hips were revised for acetabular cup–cement interface dissociation, none of which had evidence of femoral component loosening or radiolucencies >1 mm. Of the other 4 hips not revised, only 1 hip (case 29) demonstrated a 2-mm radiolucency and was considered loose.

The sensitivities and specificities for EBRA-FCA detection of migration and the known clinical outcome of femoral components were determined (Table 4). EBRA-FCA had a 44% sensitivity (95% CI: 13.6–78.7) and 65% specificity (95% CI: 40.7–84.6) at 2 years for detecting the femoral component failures, which improved to 88% sensitivity (95% CI: 51.0–99.1) and 75% specificity (95% CI: 50.8–91.3) over the duration of latest follow-up.

Migration patterns with respect to femoral head migration or stem tip migration were evaluated at the 2-year and latest follow-up (Table 5, see Fig. 1). Because the definition of migration was any migration detected by EBRA-FCA >2 mm, the migration patterns were divided into four groups: (1) femoral head and stem tip migration <2 mm; (2) femoral head migration only (femoral head >2 mm, stem tip <2 mm); (3) stem tip migration only (femoral head <2 mm, stem tip >2 mm); and (4) femoral head and stem tip migration >2 mm.

In addition, to correlate migration patterns in terms of clinical function, three clinical groups were formed: hips revised, hips that became loose, and hips not loose/functioning well at latest follow-up. The absolute change in maximum migration at the femoral head or stem tip at 2 years and at latest follow-up was measured. A significant difference between the three groups ($P = 0.025$) was found. A paired t test was done using SIDAK to adjust for multiple comparisons; the difference lied mainly between hips functioning well and those with stem lucencies >1 mm ($P = 0.022$), whereas there was no significant difference between the functioning-well group and the revision group ($P = 0.991$). Thus, the migration at 2 years remains high but steady for the revision group, low but steady for the clinical functioning-well group, and varied for the stem lucency group, which has not been revised.

Discussion

EBRA-FCA successfully detected early 2-year migration in 11 of the 29 hips studied and correlated clinically with three of the femoral failures requiring revision surgery at an average of 87.6 months (range, 81–93 months). These three revisions (cases 1–3) were within group I-A and were considered loose, along with another hip (case 4) that had significant migration of the femoral head and stem tip and an associated radiolucency of 3 mm. The other hip (case 5) within group I-A, which is clinically functional at 119.5 months and did not demonstrate any radiolucencies, showed significant femoral head migration (3.08 mm at 2 years and 3.38 mm at latest follow-up) but no stem tip migration and was considered stable. This finding may indicate measurement error or secondary stabilization. The fourth revision (case 6), within group I-B, showed significant migration at 2 years; however, no migration at latest follow-up (71 months) and no radiolucencies were demonstrated. The femoral component was well fixed during implant retrieval analysis. With the remaining 5 hips in group I-B showing no migration at latest follow-up, no associated radiolucencies, and being clinically functional at an average 95.8 months (range, 89–103 months), the authors believe that this may represent secondary stabilization of the femoral component or measurement error. In reviewing the migration patterns of group I-B, 3 hips (cases 8, 9, and 11) demonstrated femoral head and stem tip migration >2 mm at 2 years and then stabilized with no migration at latest follow-up, whereas 3 hips (cases 6,7, and 10) demonstrated femoral head migration at 2 years but then demonstrated no migration at latest follow-up, which may represent measurement error (see Fig. 1).

Within group II-A, EBRA-FCA detected no migration at 2 years but detected migration at an average of 92.8 months of follow-up in 8 hips. Two of these hips (cases 18 and 19) were revised at an average of 118.5 months, and the femoral components were found to be loose and associated with radiolucencies >1 mm. Implant retrieval analysis demonstrated disruption of the cement–bone interface with granulomatis-like soft tissue filling the bony voids throughout the head. In addition, EBRA-FCA began detecting the migration after 2 years and continues to track migration with continued follow-up and thus represents the ability of EBRA to detect late migration of the femoral component and probable late loosening and failure within this group. Only 2 additional hips are associated with radiolucencies >1 mm and considered loose. The remaining 4 hips are associated with no radiolucencies and need to be closely monitored to correlate outcome because EBRA-FCA demonstrates migration before radiolucencies show up on radiographs [14]. In 10 hips, EBRA-FCA detected no significant migration (group II-B). All 6 revisions had a well-fixed femoral component with no migration as analyzed by EBRA-FCA. The remaining 4 hips are clinically functional at an average 90 months; however, 1 hip has a 2-mm radiolucency and is considered loose.

This series of cemented hip resurfacings was a challenging series to analyze due to its small size and the different combinations of fixation used [18]. The main mode of failure was predominantly the cemented acetabular component, which may have led to some rotational differences detected as migration by EBRA-FCA. In addition, many of the patients did not undergo any standardized radiographic follow-up, which may have contributed to radiograph incompatibility and rejection by the EBRA-FCA software. Looking at the change in maximum migration at 2 years and at latest follow-up, however, there were significant differences between the three groups based on their clinical function. Using this analysis, the different types of migration patterns can be appreciated: some hips that were probably stable eventually became loose (group II-A) and other hips that exhibited some motion stabilized and continue to function well (group I-B). In addition, the increasing sensitivity and specificity at latest follow-up indicate a surveillance function to allow prediction of failure at an intermediate or longer-term date.

These observations and trends in migration patterns (see Fig. 1) are encouraging for the use of EBRA-FCA to monitor metal-on-metal hip resurfacing; however, a larger sample size is required to further define and validate the ability of EBRA-FCA to provide early detection and surveillance for femoral component loosening. Of the 29 hips analyzed in this study, the EBRA software only accepted 53% of the radiographs scanned versus 80% from other series [9,14,17]. Further prospective planning and the need for reproducible radiographs in a larger group of patients will provide more support for the following guidelines in the analysis of femoral component migration in hip resurfacing:

1. Femoral head and stem tip migration <2 mm represents no migration.
2. Femoral head migration only (femoral head >2 mm, stem tip <2 mm) most likely represents no migration and may be a result of rotational differences on the radiographs or measurement error. As indicated previously, further studies are needed to define a cutoff point for critical head migration.
3. Femoral head migration <2 mm and stem tip migration >2 mm most likely represents loosening. The femoral head may have moved within the plane of the radiograph so that EBRA did not detect the movement.
4. Femoral head and stem tip migration >2 mm represents loosening.

Acknowledgments

The authors thank Fred Dorey for his assistance in the statistical analysis. The authors would like to acknowledge that these patients were operated on by Harlan C. Amstutz, MD. The authors graciously acknowledge support from the McGowen Foundation.

References

[1] Daniel J, Pynsent PB, McMinn DJ. Metal-on-metal resurfacing of the hip in patients under the age of 55 years with osteoarthritis. J Bone Joint Surg Br 2004; 86(2):177–84.

[2] McMinn D, Treacy R, Lin K, et al. Metal on metal surface replacement of the hip. Experience of the McMinn prothesis. Clin Orthop 1996;329(Suppl):89–98.

[3] Eisler T, Svensson O, Muren C, et al. Early loosening of the stemmed McMinn cup. J Arthroplasty 2001; 16(7):871–6.

[4] Schmalzried TP, Fowble VA, Ure KJ, et al. Metal on metal surface replacement of the hip. Technique, fixation, and early results. Clin Orthop 1996;329(Suppl): S106–14.

[5] Amstutz HC, Beaule PE, Dorey FJ, et al. Metal-on-metal hybrid surface arthroplasty: two to six-year follow-up study. J Bone Joint Surg Am 2004;86(1): 28–39.

[6] Beaule PE, Amstutz HC. Surface arthroplasty of the hip revisited: current indications and surgical technique. In: Sinha RJ, editor. Hip replacement trends and controversies. New York: Marcel Dekker; 2002. p. 261–97.

[7] McKellop H, Amstutz HC, Lu B, et al. A hip simulator study of the wear of large diameter, metal-on-metal hip surface replacements. 27th Annual Meeting Transactions, 2001. Minneapolis (MN): Society for Biomaterials; 2001. p. 339.

[8] Mjoberg B. Theories of wear and loosening in hip prostheses. Wear-induced loosening vs loosening-induced wear—a review. Acta Orthop Scand 1994; 65(3):361–71.

[9] Krismer M, Biedermann R, Stockl B, et al. The prediction of failure of the stem in THR by measurement of early migration using EBRA-FCA. Einzel-Bild-Roentgen-Analyse-femoral component analysis. J Bone Joint Surg Br 1999;81(2):273–80.

[10] Freeman MA, Plante-Bordeneuve P. Early migration and late aseptic failure of proximal femoral prostheses. J Bone Joint Surg Br 1994;76(3):432–8.

[11] Walker PS, Mai SF, Cobb AG, et al. Prediction of clinical outcome of THR from migration measurements on standard radiographs. A study of cemented Charnley and Stanmore femoral stems. J Bone Joint Surg Br 1995;77(5):705–14.

[12] Ilchmann T, Markovic L, Joshi A, et al. Migration and wear of long-term successful Charnley total hip replacements. J Bone Joint Surg Br 1998;80(3):377–81.

[13] Kobayashi A, Donnelly WJ, Scott G, et al. Early radiological observations may predict the long-term survival of femoral hip prostheses. J Bone Joint Surg Br 1997;79(4):583–9.

[14] Beaule PE, Krismer M, Mayrhofer P, et al. EBRA-FCA for measurement of migration of the femoral component in surface arthroplasty of the hip. J Bone Joint Surg Br, in press.

[15] Selvik G. Roentgen stereophotogrammetry. A method for the study of the kinematics of the skeletal system. Acta Orthop Scand Suppl 1989;232:1–51.

[16] Karrholm J, Herberts P, Hultmark P, et al. Radiostereometry of hip prostheses. Review of methodology and clinical results. Clin Orthop 1997;344:94–110.

[17] Biedermann R, Krismer M, Stockl B, et al. Accuracy of EBRA-FCA in the measurement of migration of femoral components of total hip replacement. Einzel-Bild-Rontgen-Analyse-femoral component analysis. J Bone Joint Surg Br 1999;81(2):266–72.

[18] Beaule PE, Le DM, Campbell P, et al. Metal-on-metal surface arthroplasty with a cemented femoral component: a 7–10 year follow-up study. J Arthroplasty 2004;19(8 Suppl 3):17–22.

[19] Amstutz HC, Thomas BJ, Jinnah R, et al. Treatment of primary osteoarthritis of the hip. A comparison of total joint and surface replacement arthroplasty. J Bone Joint Surg Am 1984;66(2):228–41.

[20] Beaule PE, Dorey FJ, LeDuff M, et al. Risk factors affecting outcome of metal-on-metal surface arthroplasty of the hip. Clin Orthop 2004;418:87–93.

[21] Howie DW, Cornish BL, Vernon-Roberts B. Resurfacing hip arthroplasty. Classification of loosening and the role of prosthesis wear particles. Clin Orthop 1990; 255:144–59.

ELSEVIER
SAUNDERS

Orthop Clin N Am 36 (2005) 251–254

ORTHOPEDIC
CLINICS
OF NORTH AMERICA

Index

Note: Page numbers of article titles are in **boldface** type.

Changing Your Address?

Make sure your subscription changes too! When you notify us of your new address, you can help make our job easier by including an exact copy of your Clinics label number with your old address (see illustration below.) This number identifies you to our computer system and will speed the processing of your address change. Please be sure this label number accompanies your old address and your corrected address—you can send an old Clinics label with your number on it or just copy it exactly and send it to the address listed below.

We appreciate your help in our attempt to give you continuous coverage. Thank you.

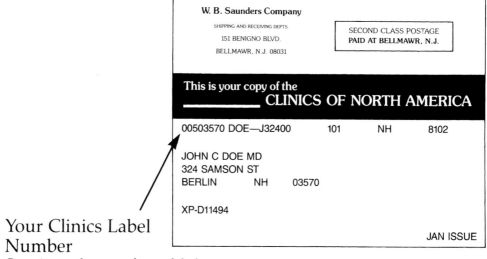

W. B. Saunders Company

SHIPPING AND RECEIVING DEPTS.
151 BENIGNO BLVD.
BELLMAWR, N.J. 08031

SECOND CLASS POSTAGE
PAID AT BELLMAWR, N.J.

This is your copy of the
_____ CLINICS OF NORTH AMERICA

00503570 DOE—J32400   101   NH   8102

JOHN C DOE MD
324 SAMSON ST
BERLIN   NH   03570

XP-D11494

JAN ISSUE

Your Clinics Label Number
Copy it exactly or send your label
along with your address to:
W.B. Saunders Company, Customer Service
Orlando, FL 32887-4800
Call Toll Free 1-800-654-2452

Please allow four to six weeks for delivery of new subscriptions and for processing address changes.

Practice, Current, Hardbound:
SATISFACTION GUARANTEED

YES! Please start my subscription to the **CLINICS** checked below with the ❑ first issue of the calendar year or ❑ current issues. If not completely satisfied with my first issue, I may write "cancel" on the invoice and return it within 30 days at no further obligation.

Please Print:

Name _____

Address_____

City_____ State _____ ZIP _____

Method of Payment
❑ Check (payable to **Elsevier**; add the applicable sales tax for your area)

❑ VISA   ❑ MasterCard   ❑ AmEx   ❑ Bill me

Card number _____ Exp. date _____

Signature _____

Staple this to your purchase order to expedite delivery

Order your subscription today. Simply complete and detach this card and drop it in the mail to receive the best clinical information in your field.

❑ **Adolescent Medicine Clinics**
❑ Individual $95
❑ Institutions $133
❑ *In-training $48

❑ **Anesthesiology**
❑ Individual $175
❑ Institutions $270
❑ *In-training $88

❑ **Cardiology**
❑ Individual $170
❑ Institutions $266
❑ *In-training $85

❑ **Chest Medicine**
❑ Individual $185
❑ Institutions $285

❑ **Child and Adolescent Psychiatry**
❑ Individual $175
❑ Institutions $265
❑ *In-training $88

❑ **Critical Care**
❑ Individual $165
❑ Institutions $266
❑ *In-training $83

❑ **Dental**
❑ Individual $150
❑ Institutions $242

❑ **Emergency Medicine**
❑ Individual $170
❑ Institutions $263
❑ *In-training $85
    ❑ Send CME info

❑ **Facial Plastic Surgery**
❑ Individual $199
❑ Institutions $300

❑ **Foot and Ankle**
Individual $160
Institutions $232

❑ **Gastroenterology**
❑ Individual $190
❑ Institutions $276

❑ **Gastrointestinal Endoscopy**
❑ Individual $190
❑ Institutions $276

❑ **Hand**
❑ Individual $205
❑ Institutions $319

❑ **Heart Failure (NEW in 2005!)**
❑ Individual $99
❑ Institutions $149
❑ *In-training $49

❑ **Hematology/Oncology**
❑ Individual $210
❑ Institutions $315

❑ **Immunology & Allergy**
❑ Individual $165
❑ Institutions $266

❑ **Infectious Disease**
❑ Individual $165
❑ Institutions $272

❑ **Clinics in Liver Disease**
❑ Individual $165
❑ Institutions $234

❑ **Medical**
❑ Individual $140
❑ Institutions $244
❑ *In-training $70
    ❑ Send CME info

❑ **MRI**
❑ Individual $190
❑ Institutions $290
❑ *In-training $95
    ❑ Send CME info

❑ **Neuroimaging**
❑ Individual $190
❑ Institutions $290
❑ *In-training $95
    ❑ Send CME inf0

❑ **Neurologic**
❑ Individual $175
❑ Institutions $275

❑ **Obstetrics & Gynecology**
❑ Individual $175
❑ Institutions $288

❑ **Occupational and Environmental Medicine**
❑ Individual $120
❑ Institutions $166
❑ *In-training $60

❑ **Ophthalmology**
❑ Individual $190
❑ Institutions $325

❑ **Oral & Maxillofacial Surgery**
❑ Individual $180
❑ Institutions $280
❑ *In-training $90

❑ **Orthopedic**
❑ Individual $180
❑ Institutions $295
❑ *In-training $90

❑ **Otolaryngologic**
❑ Individual $199
❑ Institutions $350

❑ **Pediatric**
❑ Individual $135
❑ Institutions $246
❑ *In-training $68
    ❑ Send CME info

❑ **Perinatology**
❑ Individual $155
❑ Institutions $237
❑ *In-training $78
    ❑ Send CME inf0

❑ **Plastic Surgery**
❑ Individual $245
❑ Institutions $370

❑ **Podiatric Medicine & Surgery**
❑ Individual $170
❑ Institutions $266

❑ **Primary Care**
❑ Individual $135
❑ Institutions $223

❑ **Psychiatric**
❑ Individual $170
❑ Institutions $288

❑ **Radiologic**
❑ Individual $220
❑ Institutions $331
❑ *In-training $110
    ❑ Send CME info

❑ **Sports Medicine**
❑ Individual $180
❑ Institutions $277

❑ **Surgical**
❑ Individual $190
❑ Institutions $299
❑ *In-training $95

❑ **Thoracic Surgery (formerly Chest Surgery)**
❑ Individual $175
❑ Institutions $255
❑ *In-training $88

❑ **Urologic**
❑ Individual $195
❑ Institutions $307
❑ *In-training $98
    ❑ Send CME info

*To receive in-training rate, orders must be accompanied by the name of affiliated institution, dates of residency and signature of coordinator on institution letterhead. Orders will be billed at the individual rate until proof of resident status is received.

© **Elsevier** 2005. Offer valid in U.S. only. Prices subject to change without notice.   **MO 10807 DF4176**

BUSINESS REPLY MAIL

FIRST-CLASS MAIL   PERMIT NO 7135   ORLANDO FL

POSTAGE WILL BE PAID BY ADDRESSEE

PERIODICALS ORDER FULFILLMENT DEPT
ELSEVIER
6277 SEA HARBOR DR
ORLANDO FL 32821-9816